THE PRINCIPLES AND PRACTICE OF CLINICAL TRIALS

The Editors

E. L. HARRIS
M.B., B.Ch., M.R.C.P., M.R.C.P.(Ed.)
Medical Director, Abbott Laboratories, Queenborough, Kent.
Clinical Assistant, West Kent Hospital, Maidstone.
Present appointment: Senior Medical Officer, Committee on Safety of Drugs.

J. D. FITZGERALD
M.B., B.Ch., B.Sc., M.R.C.P.(Ed.)
Research Department, I.C.I. Pharmaceuticals Division.
Department of Cardiology, Manchester Royal Infirmary,
Manchester.

Foreword by
SIR MAX ROSENHEIM
K.B.E., M.D., P.R.C.P.
Professor of Medicine, University of London.
Director of Medical Unit, University College Hospital.
President of the Royal College of Physicians, London.

The Principles
and Practice
of Clinical Trials

*Based on a Symposium organised by
the Association of Medical Advisers in the
Pharmaceutical Industry*

Edited by
E. L. HARRIS
J. D. FITZGERALD

Foreword by
SIR MAX ROSENHEIM

E. & S. LIVINGSTONE
EDINBURGH AND LONDON
1970

ISBN 0 443 00716 0

Printed in Great Britain

FOREWORD

The therapeutic revolution of the past thirty years, with the introduction of so many potent synthetic drugs, has resulted mainly from research in the laboratories of the pharmaceutical industry. Of the stream of compounds that leave the chemist's bench, few survive the long series of rigorous tests for pharmacological activity, for specificity and for animal toxicity to reach the stage of human trial. Those that then appear to be both safe and active as a result of preliminary tests in man must be submitted to the most careful clinical trial before final acceptance by the Committee on Safety of Drugs permits clinical use.

The controlled clinical trial of new therapeutic agents is a discipline that has been evolved and has become most highly developed in Great Britain and for which a rigid ethical code now exists. The organisation of such trials demands the closest cooperation between the pharmaceutical industry and the medical profession and the present friendly and effective relationship, based on mutual confidence and understanding, owes much to the work of the medical advisers to the pharmaceutical industry. These medical advisers are experts in the various techniques of controlled trial and in the statistical analysis and interpretation of results. Though not normally directly involved, they have acquired a great knowledge and understanding of the difficulties and problems that face the clinician.

As President of the Royal College of Physicians of London I was, therefore, delighted when Dr G. R. Daniel, Chairman of the Association of Medical Advisers in the Pharmaceutical Industry suggested that their association might hold a symposium on the Principles and Practice of Clinical Trials in the College. The present volume includes the many interesting contributions to that symposium—contributions from research workers in industry, from pure pharmacologists and clinical pharmacologists, from clinicians and statisticians—and presents a most fascinating and readable account of clinical trials. Illustrating as it does the close cooperation between academic and industrial scientists, I am confident that this book will receive a warm welcome and will be widely appreciated; I believe that it will contribute to the strengthening of the understanding that now so closely links the pharmaceutical industry and the medical profession.

M. L. ROSENHEIM

1970.

v

PREFACE

This book is aimed at students, new medical recruits to the pharmaceutical industry and clinicians involved in the assessment of drugs. It is based on a symposium organised by the Association of Medical Advisers in the Pharmaceutical Industry which was held at the Royal College of Physicians, London in February 1969.

Members of our Association have felt for some time that despite the availability of a number of excellent texts on statistics and clinical trial methodology, there is a need for a simple but practical guide to clinical trials.

The book is in two parts. The first deals with the principles and practice of clinical trials. Our object has been to dissect the clinical trial into its component parts and then reassemble it into a logical guide for those wishing to traverse the rock-strewn and pot-holed path of drug assessment in man. The second part presents a number of examples of how the principles and practice can be applied.

We wish to thank the participants for their ready cooperation: Dr G. Daniel, Chairman; Dr D. Burley, Treasurer; members of the Committee of A.M.A.P.I. for assistance with the organisation of the symposium; the Royal College of Physicians for help and hospitality, and the publishers, E. & S. Livingstone, for their very helpful collaboration. Special thanks to Mrs E. Mills who has shouldered much of the secretarial and co-ordinating duties.

E.L.H.

1970.　　　　　　　　　　　　　　　　　　　　　　　　　J.D.F.

CHAIRMEN

Sir Max Rosenheim, KBE, MD, PRCP. President of the Royal College of Physicians, London.

Dr. R. F. Crampton, MB, PhD, FIBiol. Director of the British Industrial Biological Research Association.

Professor M. Hamilton, MD, MRCP, DPM. Nuffield Professor of Psychiatry, University of Leeds.

Professor W. Linford Rees, MD, FRCP, DPM. Department of Psychological Medicine, St. Bartholomew's Hospital, London.

LIST OF CONTRIBUTORS

T. B. Binns, FRCP, MRCP, DCH. Director of Clinical Research, CIBA Laboratories Ltd.

D. M. Burley, MB, BCh., MRCS. Medical Department, CIBA Laboratories Ltd.

D. R. Chambers, MB, DRCOG, LLB. Head of Department of Clinical Investigation, Hoechst Pharmaceuticals Ltd.

W. I. Cranston, MD, FRCP. Professor of Medicine, St. Thomas's Hospital, London.

G. R. Daniel, MB, BA. Medical Director, E. R. Squibb & Sons Ltd.

J. G. Domenet, MB, ChB. Medical Department Geigy (U.K.) Ltd.

C. C. Downie, MD. Medical Department, Imperial Chemical Industries Ltd.

J. F. Dunne, MB, BSc. Lecturer, Department of Pharmacology & Therapeutics, London Hospital Medical College.

J. D. Fitzgerald, MB, BCh, BSc, MRCPE. Medical Department, Imperial Chemical Industries Ltd.

A. W. Galbraith, MB, DRCOG, DCH. Medical Department, Geigy (U.K.) Ltd.

E. M. Glaser, MD, MRCP, PhD, FIBiol. Director of Research and Development, Riker Laboratories.

J. A. L. Gorringe, MD, MRCPE. Director of Clinical Investigation Parke Davis & Company.

J. J. Grimshaw, BSc, FIS. Head of Statistics and Management Services, Beecham Research Laboratories.

M. Hamilton, MD, MRCP, DPM. Nuffield Professor Psychiatry, University of Leeds.

E. L. Harris, MB, MRCP, MRCPE. Medical Director, Abbott Laboratories Ltd.

C. R. B. Joyce, MA, BSc, PhD. Reader in Pharmacology, The London Hospital.

H. J. C. J. L'Etang, BM, BA, DIH. Medical Department, John Wyeth & Brother Ltd.

J. S. Malpas, D.Phil., MRCP. Senior Lecturer in Medicine, St. Bartholomew's Hospital. Consultant Physician, St. Leonard's Hospital, London.

Cyril Maxwell, MB, ChB. Medical Department, Geigy (U.K.) Ltd.

M. Shepherd, DM, DPM, MRCP. Professor of Epidemiological Psychiatry, Institute of Psychiatry, University of London.

G. E. Sowton, MD, MRCP. Assistant Director, Institute of Cardiology.

D. W. Vere, MD, MRCP. Consultant Physician and Senior Lecturer, The London Hospital.

P. Wade. Senior Librarian, Royal Society of Medicine.

J. A. Waycott, MRCP, DCH. Medical Department, Imperial Chemical Industries Ltd.

CONTENTS

PART I

PRINCIPLES AND PRACTICE

PART II

PRACTICAL APPLICATION

PART I

PRINCIPLES AND PRACTICE

HISTORICAL ASPECTS OF DRUG EVALUATION

H. J. C. J. L'ETANG

Dr Bartlett, an American investigator, has emphasised that in therapeutic trials the subjects under study should be comparable as regards
race and social class, the disease in question and the treatment should
be clearly defined and there must be a correct selection of cases. If
the name of this investigator is unfamiliar you need not reproach
yourself or your technical staff. He died over 100 years ago, and
clinical trials were performed many years before his day. For this
observation, and for much of my talk, I am greatly indebted to a
comprehensive survey by Dr J. P. Bull who is at present the director
of the M.R.C. Industrial Injuries Unit at Birmingham.

The Chairman of our Association has drawn my attention to an
early clinical trial recorded in the greatest book of all; and what better
source than the book of Daniel, Chapter I. The investigation may be
as familiar to you as it was unfamiliar to me. Nebuchadnezzar II,
having invested Jerusalem and defeated the Israelis in 600 BC, took
several youths back to his own country for indoctrination and training.
They were carefully selected. All were of royal or princely blood;
social class I, in fact. All were physically fit with a high I.Q. They
were to be put on a rigid diet of meat and wine for three years with
one of the eunuchs acting as the monitor. Daniel persuaded the monitor
to give him and three others a diet of pulse and water for 10 days;
when, it is recorded, they were fairer in countenance and fatter in
body than the other subjects who were given meat and wine. Daniel
had ruined the trial, the eunuch had defied the King, and the trial had
become uncontrolled. I have searched the Book of Daniel and it is not
recorded what Nebuchadnezzar did to the eunuch.

It was not so long after biblical times, judging the passage of time
in the broad perspective of history, that the essential qualities of a
therapeutic trial were described. About AD 1000 Avicenna recommended that drugs should be tried on opposed cases and he stressed
the importance of human pharmacology when he warned ' that testing
a drug on a lion or a horse might not prove anything about its effect
on man '.

In view of this profound statement Bull first asks why advances
in therapeutic trials did not occur until the nineteenth and twentieth
centuries and then goes far to answer these questions by citing six
adverse factors that delayed progress: (1) reverence for authority in
medicine, (2) ethical considerations involved in the doctor/patient
relationship, (3) poor records, due originally to lack of printing, (4) lack

3

of investigational facilities, (5) polypharmacy and (6) lack of active remedies.

I suggest that the first five conditions are still with us today but that the sixth—lack of active remedies—has largely been solved by the research and development in the pharmaceutical industry; an activity that has brought abuse rather than praise from certain authorities.

One of the first recorded, if not the first, therapeutic trial had the virtue and the genius of simplicity. In 1600 four ships had been sent to India by the East India Company and, for some unstated reason, one had been provided with lemon juice as part of the rations; this crew was free from scurvy. Our profession is sceptical and conservative and it was not for another 147 years that James Lind initiated his classic therapeutic trial on 12 patients with similar signs of scurvy: 2 were given cider as a dietary supplement, 2 vitriol, 2 vinegar, 2 oranges and lemons and the remainder a mixture, and one is fearful of its content, prepared by a hospital surgeon.

It is obvious to us now that the results emphasised the prophylactic value of oranges and lemons but Lind was not immediately convinced and lemon juice was not issued regularly for another 50 years. It should make us wonder whether any of our own therapeutic trials—discarded as negative or inconclusive—actually have merit which will be discovered by our successors.

Using the analogy of the monkey and the typewriter it was only a matter of time before accurate clinical entities were described and something approaching a satisfactory treatment was selected from a multitude of remedies. Infectious diseases provided admirable tests for therapy, for alterations or improvement could be reasonably compared with the immediate, and usually high, mortality. Inoculation against smallpox was tried in six convicts in 1721. The Sovereign's permission had to be obtained but I cannot discover if consent was sought from the subjects. In the last years of the eighteenth century Jenner and Pearson described clinical trials in patients who showed immunity to smallpox inoculation after a previous attack of cowpox. The purist may criticise the studies because of the small number of cases, the uncertain method of transferring infection and ignorance of any previous immunity. Precise methodology in clinical trials is a good servant but may become a bad master; we should be indulgent to those who get the right answer the wrong way.

The great advance of the therapeutic trial in the nineteenth century was encouraged by the development of statistical analysis. In 1834 Louis, discussing the effects of different methods of treatment, against different diseases in different classes of patient, wrote: ' Here again it is necessary to count. And it is, in great part at least, because hitherto this method has not been at all, or rarely employed, that the science of therapeutics is still so uncertain.'

Louis' influence was stimulating although it tended to have a negative effect: exposing the limitations of established therapy rather than demonstrating the advantages of new therapy.

Oliver Wendell Holmes exposed the fallacious approach that led to over-medication but blamed the patient who 'insists on being poisoned'. In 1865 Dr H. G. Sutton of Guy's studied 20 patients with rheumatic fever whose treatment was confined to mint water. His conclusions may still be valid: 'A perusal of the above cases tends to show that the best treatment for rheumatic fever has still to be determined.'

Technical advances in bacteriology and the preparation of vaccines permitted new methods of treatment to be assessed. The trial of Pasteur's vaccine in 1881 for the prophylaxis of anthrax in animals was rigidly controlled. The dose of inoculum was meticulously measured and administered alternately to protected and unprotected animals. Despite this scientific experiment it is understandable that the first human trials with anti-diphtheritic serum were uncontrolled; the mortality in treated patients being compared either with the previous year's mortality in the same hospital or with the current mortality in other hospitals. Fibiger, a Danish physician, presumably convinced himself that uncontrolled trials were imprecise and only treated alternate cases of diphtheria with serum, analysing the subjects for comparability in age, sex and severity. The use of serum reduced mortality but Bull has pointed out that the validity of the trial is lessened because diphtheria in 1898 was only associated with an 8 per cent mortality; a chance that may have eased any subsequent pangs of conscience on the part of this bold, but precise, investigator.

Considerable advances in the controlled clinical trial occurred in the 1920's and these have attracted little attention. Their instigator was Brigadier J. A. Sinton, an intellectually outstanding but irascible personality, who formed a Malaria Treatment Centre in the Punjab. Here for the first time anti-malarial drugs were evaluated on a rational basis. So successful was he in finding the best regime that soon there were no more cases, no more trials and no treatment centre.

Sinton was later elected a Fellow of the Royal Society; a humdrum honour in comparison with the Victoria Cross which he won in Nebuchadnezzar's former Kingdom in 1916. It is said that on this occasion he lost his temper with the enemy rather than his own side.

In the same period the concept of the controlled clinical trial was disseminated in a dramatic manner to a wider public by a popular American novelist. Sinclair Lewis, the son of a doctor, wrote in collaboration with Paul de Kruit, a bacteriologist and science writer, a novel about doctors and research workers entitled *Martin Arrowsmith*. A new bacteriophage against plague was tested and Dr Arrowsmith, torn between the objective demands of scientific enquiry and his subjective concern for the patients, was unable to withhold active treatment from the controls. 700,000 copies of this book have been sold in various covers since 1925. More recently Dr John Wilson, one of the founders of this Association, has also instructed the general public through his novel entitled *The Double Blind*.

Bull has written: ' The years since 1935 have possibly seen more clinical trials than occurred in the whole of previous medical history.' It might be argued that for the first time therapeutic substances were provided in sufficient quantity and variety to make clinical trials possible. Between 1936 and 1938 the new sulphonamides were given in uncontrolled trials for the treatment of puerperal septicaemia and cerebrospinal meningitis; and in controlled trials for the treatment of erysipelas and lobar pneumonia. But another influence was lighting the way ahead. In the first half of 1937 the whole question of statistics in relation to medical problems was discussed in a series of articles by Professor Bradford Hill in the *Lancet*. Did the problems, created by the need to evaluate these exciting new remedies, create in turn a need for more precise methods of evaluation? Or did Bradford Hill, like Louis one hundred years before, make clinicians aware of the imprecision of subjective impressions? Speculation is really unprofitable because it is clear that Sir Austin, whether responding to demands or stimulating interest, played a vital role.

Nevertheless we must not forget that the Medical Research Council organised a Therapeutic Trials Committee in 1931. It should be emphasised that this was done at the request of the Association of British Chemical Manufacturers. As a result of the trials conducted by this M.R.C. Committee substances such as calciferol, digoxin, prontosil, sulphanilamide and stilboestrol eventually became available to doctors. In many trials it was possible to get objective proof of efficacy, by means of instrumental and laboratory data, so that the use of untreated control patients was avoided. Some years later untreated controls were available for the M.R.C. trials on streptomycin, PAS and isoniazid since supplies of these substances were unfortunately limited.

If we look back on nearly 1,000 years of clinical trials we must be impressed by the frequency with which lessons have been learned, forgotten, re-learned and discarded; and we must be saddened how methods, that might have selected potent drugs for the relief of suffering, have lain buried for centuries. Lest we are guilty in our generation of these sins of omission and commission we should both remember and try to disprove the cynical statement: 'All we learn from history is that we don't learn from history.'

REFERENCES

BULL, J. P. (1959). The historical development of clinical therapeutic trials. *J. chron. Dis.* **10**, 218.

GREEN, F. H. K. (1954). The clinical evaluation of remedies. *Lancet*, **2**, 1085.

NATURAL HISTORY OF A TYPICAL DRUG

E. L. HARRIS

It is impossible to generalise on the natural history of a drug because they have entered therapeutics in many varied ways. Perhaps we should start by defining a drug. What better definition than that adopted by the Committee on Safety of Drugs (1968), namely 'Any substance or mixture of substances destined for administration to man for use in the diagnosis, treatment, investigation or prevention of disease or for the modification of physiological function.'

Drugs have come to be used in therapeutics in the following ways:

1. From primitive medicine, folklore and possibly witchcraft—it is very difficult here in many cases to precisely pinpoint the origin. Good examples are the use of quinine for malaria, lime juice for scurvy and ma huang (ephedrine) for asthma.

2. The investigation of natural products, from vegetable or animal origin. Important examples from vegetable sources are reserpine, digitalis, and the various opium alkaloids. Animal sources include thyroxin, liver extract and intrinsic factor.

3. Synthesis of new chemicals around natural substances, such as the synthetic narcotic analgesics, ascorbic acid and the semi-synthetic penicillins.

4. Synthesis of new chemicals around existing drugs. At the moment this is by far the largest group of therapeutic agents. A very good example is the succession of simple chemical steps from Prontosil to the short acting, then long acting sulphonamides, carbonic anhydrase inhibitors, oral anti-diabetic agents, and the thiazide diuretics. Serendipity undoubtedly played some part in their discovery.

5. New drugs which have resulted from the scientific study of physiological and pathological processes in animals and man, for instance insulin in diabetes, cortisone in Addison's disease and the Salk vaccine in poliomyelitis.

6. Last but certainly not least, happy chance, those empirical accidents. These accidents are only recognised by the highly trained and astute. A good example is the discovery of the analgesic and anti-inflammatory properties of phenylbutazone when it was used as a solvent for amidopyrine for administration by injection. Another is the discovery of the sweetening effects of cyclamates. In 1937 a research chemist brushed some loose tobacco shreds from his lips while smoking a cigarette and to his amazement detected a sweet taste. This was enough to arouse his curiosity and he said 'Almost as a reflex action I began to taste every compound in sight. Within a minute I

knew that of the dozen or more compounds on the bench the sweet substance was the salt of N-cyclohexylsulphamic acid.'

As the majority of new therapeutic agents are developed by the pharmaceutical industry rather than by University or Government laboratories, we will discuss the genesis of a new drug in a typical firm. The great majority of new therapeutic agents have been the result of concerted work by teams consisting of chemists, biochemists, pharmacologists, pathologists, pharmacists, clinical pharmacologists and clinicians. A pattern of drug development has emerged and the various stages have become increasingly refined. Figure 1 shows graphically the progress of a drug from idea to market place.

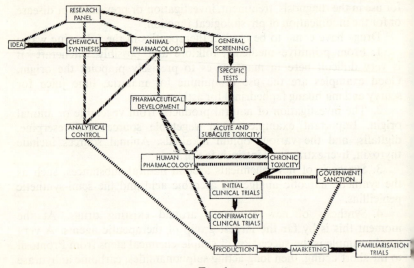

Fig. 1
The evolution of a 'typical' drug.

The first stage is that of the idea. This may originate from any source—often from a research chemist who suggests that by modifying the structure of a known compound he could possibly enhance activity, make it more specific, reduce its toxicity or increase its oral absorption. Other sources are attempts to modify naturally occurring substances or to synthesise these. The idea may originate from clinical practice, i.e. the market place, where a specific need is indicated.

Whatever the source of the idea, it is considered by a research panel consisting of medical, chemical, pharmacological, pharmaceutical and commercial interests. This panel will be responsible for the direction of research and will co-ordinate the results obtained. If the panel feel that the idea has merit, then the research chemist sets about synthesising the compound or a number of related compounds. This can be a very long and arduous task; it has been estimated that synthesis and initial biological screening of a single compound can take up to 400 man hours to achieve. Concurrently with the chemist's activity the Analytical Department tackles the problem of identification and assay of the new entity. Frequently this involves research into new chemical and biological screening methods.

When sufficient quantities have been made the pure drugs are handed over to the pharmacologist who carries out a programme of empirical screening tests, designed to cover as wide a range of pharmacological actions as economically as possible so as to expose any effects which might be of therapeutic use. If an action is detected more detailed experiments to elucidate this are carried out.

Many compounds are rejected at this stage either because of lack of activity or gross toxicity. Those that do survive are again considered by the research panel who decide whether the agent has sufficient promise to go forward to assess its safety in animals.

There are three phases in toxicity testing. The first is the acute toxicity study which deals with the quantitative assessment of the short term effects of a drug. The response is noted after a single oral or parenteral dose, or several doses given within 24 hours. These tests are carried out in a variety of species.

The next is sub-acute toxicity, and in general covers repeated dosage in at least two species, such as mice and rats, for periods up to 90 days. An additional non-rodent species, e.g. dog, is often included.

Chronic studies are for the duration of life in the animal—rats and mice are suitable. Occasionally long term studies are employed in other animals such as dogs and monkeys for periods up to two years.

The precise protocol varies with each drug. An action relevant to that intended in man should be shown in at least one species. Also the absorption, excretion and metabolism of the drug are examined as well as effects on fertility and reproduction.

At these early stages Pharmaceutical Development enters the picture because they are responsible for the presentation of the drug both to the pharmacologist and to the toxicologist. Drug activity may be very significantly altered by the formulation in which it is made available. To take just a few examples of how physical manipulation can change the properties of a drug, a reduction in particle size by increasing total surface area of the drug can produce up to fourfold increase in absorption as has been shown with such agents as griseofulvin and spironolactone. Neomycin which is frequently formulated with kaolin, unless properly compounded, may become strongly adsorbed reducing its antibacterial activity.

When the exacting toxicological studies are completed and the Research Panel is satisfied with all the data that has been generated, the drug is administered to healthy volunteers. This is the stage of clinical pharmacology which sets out to answer—is this drug absorbed, metabolised and excreted in man as in animals, does it have a pharmacological action and is it safe for further study in man?

When these studies have been satisfactorily completed, the drug has then to be assessed in patients. In the majority of countries before this can be done a submission must be made to a central Government organisation, in the U.K. the Committee on Safety of Drugs. They will consider the chemistry, pharmacology, toxicity and clinical pharmacological studies and, if satisfied, sanction the early clinical trials.

If clinical trials show that a drug has a definite place, the Company will wish to place it on the market. Government sanction to do so must again be obtained. Process chemists and engineers now apply themselves to producing bulk supplies of the drug, initially using a pilot plant and later on full production facilities. At the same time pharmacists scale up the production of the formulation, and all the many other activities such as packaging, labelling and literature preparation are set in motion.

At this stage it is important to emphasise one aspect of developing a new drug, namely the enormous cost involved. To illustrate this point, a team consisting of two chemists, two biologists and a biochemist, researching a new therapeutic substance, along with all their equipment and ancillary scientists and technical staff, would cost approximately £130,000 per annum. In order to get the problem in perspective, it is estimated that only one out of approximately 3,000 drugs researched will eventually survive.

REFERENCES

CHEMICAL AND ENGINEERING NEWS (1966). The story of cyclamates. *Chem. Engng News,* **44,** 114.

COMMITTEE ON SAFETY OF DRUGS (1968). Notes for the guidance of manufacturers and other persons developing or proposing to market a drug in the United Kingdom, p. 3.

THE PHASES OF THE CLINICAL TRIAL

E. L. Harris

A good introduction to the subject of clinical trials is Schneiderman's (1961): 'Clinical trials are seductive. Following the soft beckoning glance, the clinician is captured in his first careless rapture. The reason for the seductiveness is clear. It seems as if any competent clinician could do them. There's no hard mathematics. There's no esoteric chemistry. There's usually little need for complicated equipment that isn't already around. And clinical trials are " research ".'

We must initially define a valid clinical trial. The best definition is that of Bradford Hill (1966), namely 'A carefully and ethically designed experiment with the aim of answering some precisely framed question '.

The steps in carrying out a clinical trial are clearly illustrated by means of a flow chart (Fig. 1). This has the advantage not only of presenting graphically the various steps involved but also allowing for an analysis of events so that if time is to be saved the critical events determining this can be shortened if possible. In the figure the lines represent activity, the circles or nodes represent an event and the figures below the activity show the length of time in days for that activity. The first phase is information retrieval and reading. It is necessary here to know all about the drug, about the pharmacological and toxicological action of various controls that can be used in the study and how other investigators have tackled the problem. The more time spent at this early stage, the more successful will be the outcome of the trial.

Activity O, in this example, would be the educational background and experience of the clinician conducting the clinical trial.

The next step is to design the trial so that it answers the precisely framed question. This would be the ideal trial into which have to be incorporated various practical and other considerations. Very briefly these include statistical advice, ethical considerations, costing, technical feasibility, clinical facilities available, pharmaceutical problems, the competence of the proposed investigators and legal considerations. When these have been incorporated into the initial design, one or more final designs are drawn up. It is possible that at this stage there are too many insuperable problems for the trial to proceed but assuming that a satisfactory protocol has been devised a decision to proceed is made and the wheels are set in motion—Activity 7.

Test medication and control drugs are ordered, manufactured and packed. Special recording apparatus may have to be obtained and frequently report forms, either for the patient or doctor, must be designed, ordered and printed. While all this is going on the clinician

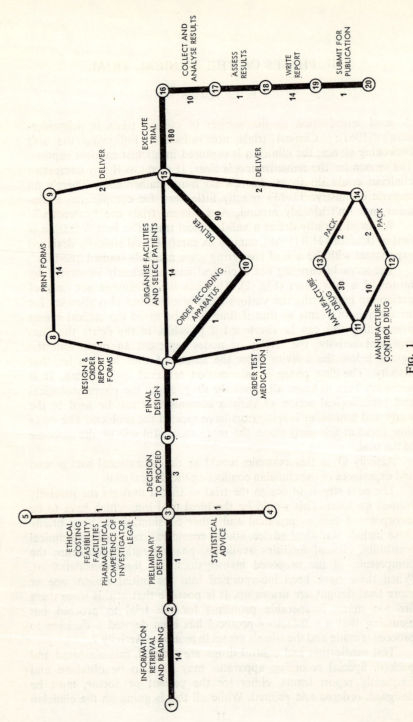

Fig. 1
Flow chart—the clinical trial

will inform his colleagues about the trial, select suitable patients according to the trial protocol and, in some cases, recruit additional staff. When all the trial material has been checked, it is forwarded to the clinician who then carries out the study in accordance with the agreed protocol.

The execution of the trial is the most important phase, is time consuming and requires close liaison between the clinician and the Medical Adviser who acts as a co-ordinator.

When the trial has been completed, all the data are collected and transposed either on to analysis sheets, punch cards or computer tape, for detailed analysis. Results from other trials using the same protocol can be incorporated at this stage.

Now the statistician again enters the picture for his interpretation of the results. He will work out whether various treatments differ significantly and will quantify this difference.

The next important phase is the assessment of results. This really is the clinician's assessment of the trial findings because whilst the statistician can work out levels of significance (perhaps one should include non-significance as well), the clinician, because of his overall knowledge, is the only one who can really make a valid judgement as to whether the aims and objects of the trial have been achieved.

The writing of a report on the trial and the results is the next phase. There is no need to emphasise how important it is that no relevant information in the trial protocol, execution and method of analysis is omitted.

The final stage is the preparation of a paper for publication. Unfortunately many manuscripts will be rejected by editorial boards and will never appear in print.

Critical path analysis can be utilised in clinical trial planning. It is defined as a method for attempting to determine the completion date for a task, taking into account all the activities which are involved.

The critical path in the figure given is indicated by the thick line, this shows the time required to complete the trial. Other activities in parallel are completed in less time and to shorten the overall duration it is obvious, in this example, that the delivery time for the recording apparatus must be improved. If this is reduced then the next limitation will be the time taken to manufacture the test medication.

Briefly clinical trials can be classified into three broad groups:

1. Initial trials—After careful assessment in normal volunteers, the drug is given to patients for the first time, to establish therapeutic efficacy and safety.

2. Confirmatory trials—Extensions of the initial trial in which larger numbers of patients are included, together with a greater range of assessments such as comparison with other therapeutic agents, other indications and different population groups.

3. Familiarisation trials—Extensions of confirmatory trials, their object being to make a larger number of clinicians familiar with the new therapeutic agent, and increase the exposure of patients to the drug—a further phase of human toxicity under more varied conditions. An offshoot of this group is sometimes known as ' promotional trials '. These trials may be controlled or uncontrolled and on the whole are carried out by less research-orientated doctors.

The brief account of the natural history of a drug and the phases of a clinical trial serve as an introduction and provide the windows which will be dressed in the following pages.

REFERENCES

HARRIS, E. L. (1966). The clinical trial in general practice. *J. Coll. gen. Practit.* **12,** 43.

HILL, A. BRADFORD (1966). *The Principles of Medical Statistics,* 8th ed. London: Lancet.

LOCKYER, K. G. (1965). *An Introduction to Critical Path Analysis.* London: Pitman.

SCHNEIDERMAN, M. A. (1961). Controlled clinical trials: Monday's count-down for Tuesday's launching. *J. new Drugs,* **1,** 250.

CLINICAL PHARMACOLOGY

Colin C. Downie

I have been given the most ill-defined title of the symposium judged by the number of attempts that have been made during the past year or two to define clinical pharmacology with any precision. I neither have the time at my disposal nor the inclination to initiate further discussion on this controversial topic; but I shall make one or two general comments to put the area on which I have chosen to speak in some sort of perspective.

Clinical pharmacology has been divided into three parts. Firstly there is the investigation of how the human subject handles a drug in terms of absorption, distribution, metabolism and excretion. Secondly there is the investigation of how the drug affects the body systems. The third part is the study of the value of the drug in the treatment of disease and its comparison with the standard method of treatment if there is one. Some argue that this latter type of investigation is not strictly within the bounds of clinical pharmacology and I will take advantage of this opinion to exclude any discussion of this aspect of drug evaluation from my presentation.

Thus in simple terms I am left with effect of the body on the drug and the drug on the body. I would like to select the first of these as being more amenable to generalisations applicable to most new compounds, whereas the second is dependent on the known biological activity of the compound.

By this far from subtle process of elimination I have narrowed my presentation to a discussion of clinical pharmacokinetics and by so doing have conformed with the present-day demand for super-specialisation accompanied by appropriate nomenclature.

The first administration to man of a new chemical is the biggest single step in the evolution of a new drug, and in many cases the step is taken with the least amount of relevant information to guide the investigator in his task. It is also the point in time when there is the greatest potential hazard to the volunteer or patient. I stress the word potential as by skill or good fortune or both the practical hazard to the human subject at this stage of drug investigation has been minimal in the past. If we are to maintain this record I believe every effort should be made to pass through this stage with all speed. Before anyone misinterprets that remark let me say that speed in this context refers to the rapid accumulation of as much data as possible with the minimal exposure of the volunteers or patients to the drug. This can only be accomplished by detailed planning of the investigation and is largely dependent upon the extent and quality of the information available from the previous experiments in animals.

Although it may appear as a digression, I should like to spend a minute or two on the subject of the studies in animals because available information from these will virtually dictate the pattern of the first investigation in man. If one were to make a list of requirements for information over and above that obtained by standard pharmacological and toxicological testing I would include the following:

1. A method for the estimation of the compound in the blood and other body fluids, preferably a chemical method but one might have to be content with a biological method.

2. A knowledge of blood levels achieved by single and multiple dosing by the appropriate routes of administration in a number of animal species.

3. An indication of the blood level at which the desirable therapeutic or pharmacological effects were observed and at which toxic signs appeared—on the premise that it is more meaningful to compare species by blood concentration rather than by other means.

4. A knowledge of the distribution, metabolism, and route of elimination of the compound.

One can, of course, prolong the list, but I do not think that would be a useful exercise at this point.

Armed with this information it is possible to plan the first investigation in man with the minimum danger to the human subjects. I mention it here only for the sake of completeness that following the administration of the drug the responses of the human subject must be monitored together with the relevant biochemical and haematological examinations at selected intervals. The interpretation of the results of these tests is simpler and more meaningful if samples are taken before the drug is given. Although it seems so obvious it is surprising how often this sample is omitted and the reasons given for the omission are often even more surprising. I will not refer to this subject again but ask you to assume that this monitoring is a continuous process throughout the early investigation of a new drug.

I feel at this stage that my purpose would be best served if I used our experience with two compounds to illustrate the points I wish to make.

The first compound I have chosen was shown in animals to have analgesic and anti-inflammatory activity by a variety of tests in a number of animal species. The toxicity tests only revealed the ulcerogenic effects at high blood levels common to all the known anti-inflammatory compounds. The clinical evaluation of the compound was free to start.

The requirements for information from pharmacodynamic studies I mentioned earlier had been met. Thus a chemical method for estimating the level of the compound in blood and urine was developed and blood levels achieved by single and multiple dosing were known. The blood levels at which both therapeutic and toxic effects were observed were documented for each species.

These findings can be summarised:

1. The compound is bound to the serum proteins.

2. The half-life in the serum varied from 3 hours in monkeys to 40 hours in rats.

3. Anti-inflammatory activity is associated with a serum level of 50 to 100 μg/ml.

4. Levels greater than 250 μg/ml were often associated with side-effects in the most susceptible species. Levels of 600 μg/ml were achieved without side-effects in monkeys.

The first studies in man were made to enable the pharmacokinetic properties to be defined and related to those found in animals. At first single doses were given, the dose being increased in the absence of any toxic effects. Blood samples were taken at 0, 3, 7, 24, 48, 72 and 96 hours. At the end of this part of the study the accumulated data is summarised in Table I.

TABLE I

Volunteers. Blood levels following single doses

Number of subjects	Dose (mg)	Maximum serum concentration (μg/ml)	Serum half-life (hours)
7	100	13·6	25
7	150-200	25·9	25·5
3	400	55·2	23

Single doses rising from 100 mg to 400 mg were given. The serum half-life lies in the region of 25 hours and the maximum serum concentration is closely related to the dose, as can be seen when the results are plotted, maximum concentration against dose showing a linear relationship (Fig. 1). From the graph it is possible to derive the figure of 9·3 μg/ml as a maximum level from a single dose of 1 mg/kg.

The next step is to look at multiple dosing at varying daily dose levels.

Doses of 50 to 400 mg daily in two divided doses were given and serum concentration is shown at 7 and 19 days (Table II). A linear relationship to the daily dose is again seen but the half-life is perhaps a little longer when measured under these circumstances, being on average in the region of 28 hours as opposed to 25 hours after single dosing.

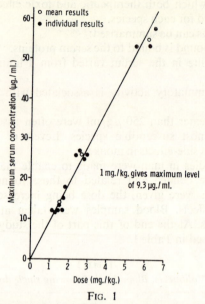

FIG. 1

The relationship between maximum serum concentration and oral dose.

TABLE II

Volunteers. Blood levels after multiple doses

Dose (twice daily)		No. of doses	Serum concentration after dose No.:		Half-life after last dose (hours)
mg	mg/kg		7	19	
25	0·4	19	10·1	8·9	
50	0·6	19	19·2	21·7	
100	1·3	20	42·6	72·1	28
150	1·7	7	70·0		34
200	3·0	7	94·5		22

With a drug with a half-life of this order it is necessary to know the rate at which the serum concentration rises to the maximum and to confirm that the level reaches equilibrium and fails to rise further. Figure 2 shows the serum levels at intervals in three subjects taking 25, 50 and 100 mg twice daily. The slow rise is seen in each case and the maximum is reached between the seventh and ninth doses, that is on the third or fourth day of treatment. Thereafter the serum level remains constant although further confirmation is required that this is so after weeks or months of dosing. In one subject blood levels were followed after dosing ceased giving a half-life of 28 hours.

Dose given in tablet form every 12 hrs.

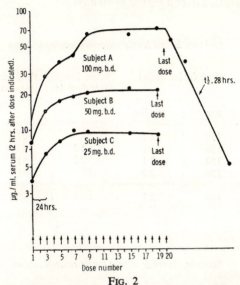

FIG. 2

The serum levels achieved by multiple dosing at three different dose levels.

It so happens that the findings I have presented so far were obtained from studies in normal human subjects. I must interpose here that it does not follow by implication that volunteers are necessary or indeed desirable for the initial studies. Each drug and each set of circumstances must be judged on their own merits. But having carried out such studies as I have described it is essential that they be repeated, perhaps to a lesser degree, in patients for whose treatment the drug is intended. This is particularly necessary in the study of drugs which are bound to the serum proteins when they are to be given to patients with known abnormalities of the proteins.

Table III summarises the data from a few patients treated for one week. A greater variability of blood levels from a given dose of drug is apparent from comparison with the volunteers. This between-patient variability appears to be related to the half-life of the drug in the serum which, in general, tends to be longer in the patients.

The measurement of blood levels continued throughout the first clinical evaluation and a summary of the results is shown in Table IV. The mean levels at each dose on day 10 again show a linear relationship and the average half-life is in the region of 35 hours thus confirming the impression from the first study in patients that it is considerably longer than in healthy subjects. As this latter study also involved a clinical assessment it was possible to make a tentative correlation between blood level and clinical response. No side-effects appeared in these 40 patients suggesting that we had not yet reached a toxic serum concentration over a period of 10 days.

TABLE III

Patients. Blood levels following multiple doses

Dose (twice daily)		Serum levels after dose 15	Half-life (hours)
mg	mg/kg		
150	2·1	58.0	27·5
150	1·7	62·3	43
150	2·1	90·5	51
150	2·3	126	61
150	2·1	84·2	45·8

TABLE IV

Patients. Average serum levels related to dose

No. of patients	Dose (twice daily)		Serum levels day 10	Calculated half-life (hours)
	mg	mg/kg		
8	100	1·9	62	32
8	150	2·7	88	31
24	200	3·5	126	37
40				35

At this stage of the evaluation of the drug it was possible to proceed with confidence to the formal clinical appraisal of its value as a therapeutic agent. Whilst these trials are in progress opportunity should be taken to increase the pharmacokinetic understanding of the compound, particularly in terms of patient variation and long-term treatment.

May I briefly turn to the study of another compound which, amongst other properties, has the ability to reduce elevated serum cholesterol levels in the blood. This activity had been observed in animals at blood levels of the drug in the region of 50 to 100 μg/ml. At these levels the half-life of the drug is 2 to 3 days in the mouse, 9 to 10 days in the dog, and 20 to 25 days in the rat. The suggested half-life to be expected in man was 30 to 40 days. I have chosen this drug as an illustration because a half-life of this length necessitates a quite different time scale for its initial pharmacokinetic studies.

I have tried to condense the data from one human subject into a single graph (Fig. 3). Dosing commenced at 20 mg per day at a time when the serum cholesterol was 350 mg per cent. The level of the drug slowly increased to reach equilibrium after four months at a level of 110 μg/ml. The cholesterol level fell during the first month and tended to stabilise at a blood level of the drug of 55 μg/ml and higher levels produced only a small further fall in serum cholesterol.

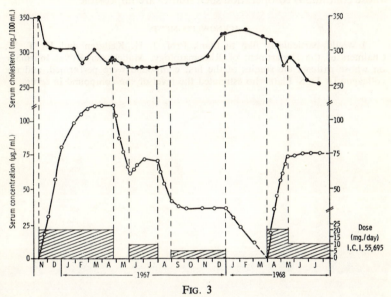

FIG. 3

The effect of different oral doses of ICI 55,695 on the serum concentration of the drug O——O and the serum cholesterol ●——●.

Once the blood level had stabilised, dosing was stopped and recommenced at a daily level of 10 mg achieving a blood level in the region of 70 μg/ml. The response of the serum cholesterol was retained. The compound was withdrawn again and recommenced at 5 mg per day. The blood level achieved by this dose stabilised at 35 μg/ml but it was apparent that the hypocholesterolaemic effect had now been lost.

The final period shown on the graph would indicate that a maintenance dose of 10 mg per day yields a blood level of 75 μg/ml and produces an optimal reduction of serum cholesterol. During the periods when the compound was withdrawn the falling blood levels were followed. The half-life was found to be in the region of 30 to 40 days, so agreeing with the prediction mentioned earlier. A similar study in two other subjects over a shorter period confirmed these findings. With this information it is possible to proceed to a formal clinical trial which will yield meaningful data quickly and with the minimum hazard to the patient.

I have attempted to show by these two examples how we have approached the task of obtaining pharmacokinetic data on new compounds. I use the word ' we ' advisedly not under any delusion of royal birth but because the accumulation of the data I have presented represents the work of many people of differing scientific disciplines without whose continuous co-operation such studies are impossible.

ACKNOWLEDGMENTS

I would particularly like to thank Prof. J. H. Kellgren and Dr T. M. Chalmers of the Department of Rheumatology, Manchester Royal Infirmary on whose patients the studies of the first compound were performed, and my colleague Dr D. S. Platt who estimated the level of the compound in serum.

ETHICAL ASPECTS OF CLINICAL TRIALS

E. M. GLASER

The nature of ethics

Ethics deal with things as they should be, not with things as they are, and ethics are based on the assumption that something can be right or wrong in itself. Ethical considerations can balance the interests of individuals and of communities. In clinical trials this is important, because the community needs knowledge and the patient needs protection. This balance is also the concern of the law. But ethics and the law are not the same. Some things are unethical but not illegal, others illegal but not unethical. Often the law enforces ethical principles.

Publications on medical ethics

There are many pronouncements on ethics of experiments on man. Among the most important of these are the code of the World Medical Association (1964), sometimes called Nuremberg Rules or Declaration of Helsinki, the directives of the Medical Research Council (1963), a report by the Royal College of Physicians (1967), and a report by a World Health Organisation Scientific Group (1968). Anyone doing research on patients or volunteers would be well advised to have some of these always at hand. Among statements by individual medical scientists some of the most interesting are those of McCance (1951), Hill (1963), and Bean (1952; 1959). To these should be added the views of a distinguished editor (Fox, 1959) and of Pope Pius XII (1952), the latter being one of a most useful pronouncement on medical ethics regardless of religious views. There is also an extensive Ciba Foundation publication on medical ethics (Wolstenholme and O'Connor, 1966) which deals largely with problems of transplantation.

New and established treatments

A clinical trial of a new treatment has much in common with any other treatment. It is important that this should be understood. Whenever we prescribe any medicine we deliberately expose the patient to the risk of discomfort or of ill effects in order to save him from worse discomfort or more serious ill effect. The risks of treatment may be small or great in relation to the risk of leaving the disease untreated, but only ineffective treatment can never go wrong. Although with modern medicaments the vast majority of patients derives benefit without harm, all therapy presupposes the balancing of advantages against disadvantages, and this is as true in clinical trials as in any other form of treatment.

23

The basic question in clinical trials of medicaments should be whether the patients in the trial are likely to benefit from it. If there is strong evidence that a new medicine has advantages over existing ones, then there can be no objections against its use. There must be satisfactory evidence of safety in relation to probable efficacy, but nowadays any new medicine is thoroughly tested on animals and volunteers, and often more is known about its toxicity and metabolism than about the established treatments with which it is compared. If the evidence about a new substance is inadequate or unfavourable, it should not be tested. If the evidence suggests that the new treatment could have advantages, it must be ethical to use it. But new substances cannot supersede existing treatments until their relative merits are proved, and it must also remain ethical to use the old treatment. It follows that if more than one treatment is justified, it is more ethical to compare them in a carefully planned trial than to choose a doubtful one (Fox, 1959; Hill, 1963; Glaser, 1964; Royal College of Physicians, 1967). Such a view was indeed expressed by Claude Bernard more than a hundred years ago. It seems reasonable to go further and to say that the patients' consent to take part in a trial is not needed if all patients are given treatments from which according to the best available knowledge they are likely to benefit (M.R.C. 1963; Glaser, 1964). This is not to say that safeguards are unnecessary, especially when a new medicine is used.

Safeguards

A medical man is always responsible for what he prescribes. But prescribing is usually influenced by what has been learnt or read, and it can be both unethical and illegal to prescribe in an eccentric manner, contrary to accepted practice. With new medicines there is no accepted practice. Thus it would be unwise for one doctor or a small team of doctors to decide what new medicines they should test and how they should do it. The patient cannot decide because he lacks expert knowledge (McCance, 1951; Fox, 1969; Hill, 1963), and he may agree in order to please his doctor, or disagree from unjustified fear. It may be wise to ask the patient, but by placing himself under medical care the patient has implied his faith in the doctor's ability to choose a treatment, and the burden of approval should rest elsewhere. It would be equally wrong for a remote bureaucratic body to make decisions about treatments (Royal College of Physicians, 1967). The best answer is probably that an intelligent and expert body should give advice after having looked at the evidence as a whole (Royal College of Physicians, 1967).

During the last four years all clinical trials of new medicines and all new uses for old ones have been approved by the Committee on Safety of Drugs as a result of a voluntary agreement. This has been an adequate safeguard which has worked well. Boards of Governors and hospital Management Committees are also increasingly sharing the responsibility of advising about clinical trials. Patients can sometimes be advised by their own doctors. More will be said about this later in connection with healthy volunteers, but with clinical trials of new medicines in hospitals the burden of arbitration can be too much to ask from a busy family practitioner, although it may be desirable to let him know. Moreover, in some clinical trials the practitioner is an experimenter. Thus the Committee on Safety of Drugs and the hospital authorities remain the best safeguards in deciding about trials from which patients are likely to benefit.

Safeguards are always necessary if a trial goes beyond what is in the patients' direct interest. For example, it may be necessary to investigate the effects of a new substance more thoroughly than the normal assessment of therapeutic effects, by frequent estimations of serum enzymes or frequent sternal punctures; or it may be necessary to perform additional gastrocopies, catheterisations, and such like. In these cases the question must be answered whether the patient is likely to suffer peril or discomfort as a result of the added investigation. If yes, he must be told what is being done, and his approval must be obtained. Obviously special approval is unnecessary for innocuous procedures like attaching e.k.g. leads, but otherwise it is better that a patient should be lost from a trial than that anyone should suffer or be at risk without his direct approval when it is not in his interest. As said before, patients cannot always judge what will be done to them. But in therapeutic trials additional tests are usually the kind of procedures which the patient has already undergone in his own interest or which can be easily explained. If for no other reason, the patients must know because it is improper that they should be deceived by their doctors.

Withholding of treatment

Patients who need treatment must get it, whether they take part in a trial or not. Untreated control groups can only be used if lack of treatment for the period contemplated is compatible with good medicine. (Sometimes the standard treatment is ineffective anyway.) Moreover, as will be said later, it is an ethical duty to do trials efficiently. It seems possible therefore to justify dummy treatments in the interest of science if this in no way conflicts with the interest of the patient. Even then it might be more honest to tell the patient that the treatment is to be scientifically assessed and that for certain periods he may get ineffective substances, or at least to tell him that he will be given substances which may or may not be effective.

If there is any likelihood of the patient's condition getting worse because treatment is withheld, and if it is really necessary in the interest of science, this can only be done if the harm is easily reversible and if the patient has agreed to it after a full explanation. The safeguard of impartial advice mentioned above must still apply.

It is sometimes considered unethical to withhold the treatment which is already in use and it is then suggested that half the patients should get the new treatment with the old, and half the old alone. As already said, a new substance should only be tested if it offers advantages. If the old treatment cannot be withheld, in many cases the new one should not be tried. If there is good reason to assume that the old and the new treatment would be good combined therapy, they should be tested together. Otherwise it can be objectionable rather than desirable to give the established treatment with the new one because such a combination could be bad medicine or it could result in a meaningless trial, both of which would be unethical.

Volunteers

Ethical problems arise when medicaments are tested on people who do not benefit from them. This is done to test undesirable side effects or normal pharmacological effects, or to study metabolites. It can be done on healthy people or on patients who happen to be in hospital for some condition unconnected with the trial. Such tests can only be done on willing subjects. What constitutes true agreement to do a test has been stated by the World Medical Association (1964). It need not be discussed here in detail because anyone with intelligence knows what is meant by doing something willingly and knowingly, and the rules are available for reference. As already said, the loss of an experimental subject is far less serious than the loss of confidence in medical research, and it is best to err on the side of caution. All those who have experience of experiments on man agree that the least common reason why a trial may go wrong is lack of cooperation from volunteers, whether they are patients or not. Here again, it is wise to seek independent advice.

Approval of a trial by the Committee on Safety of Drugs, Boards of Governors, or Management Committees is adequate advice for any trial on volunteers in hospitals. Problems can arise when new substances are tested within a pharmaceutical company.

It is a good principle that those who first take a new substance should be the people most closely connected with tests on animals. Those who decide that a new substance can be safely tried in man should have enough confidence to take it themselves. If they will not take it themselves, they should not give it to others. Those who know the most about the substance and who are the most experienced scientists can make the best personal decisions about it and they are also the best able to observe their own subjective effects. Thus the first to take a new substance might be the research director, the medical director, the senior toxicologist, or advisers in pathology. I have combined the functions of research director and medical director for several years, and I have always claimed the duty and the right of taking a new substance first, usually followed by several senior scientific colleagues. But nobody has the right to risk his own health. All those concerned must agree that the new substance can be taken by any of them. I have been overruled once by a colleague responsible for pathology who did not agree that I should take a tiny amount of a new substance. I was unconvinced, but I accepted his ruling. It might or might not have been foolish to refuse such advice, but it would have been bad medicine, bad science, and bad ethics, to go against expert advice based on the assessment of all the evidence.

It should be said in passing that the risks of taking a new substance are usually small. Toxicological tests on animals are becoming increasingly reliable. Moreover, one can gradually build up the dose with careful checks and little risk.

Systematic studies of side effects, detailed studies of metabolism, and measurements of pharmacological actions in man, can often be done on patients who benefit from the treatment. With the limitations that the therapy must be justifiable and that test needed only for research must be approved, it is reasonable that patients should help with research. Claude Bernard went further and considered this a duty. But many tests are necessary on healthy volunteers, mostly from within the company where a new substance was developed. The investigators' competence is a most important prerequisite, and a number of simple safeguards can be used (Glaser, 1964) which will be briefly considered.

A useful procedure is to obtain the volunteers' permission that their family doctor should be told about the trial. The doctor is then sent a letter which states briefly but adequately what is to be done, and the doctor is asked to advise the patient not to take part in the trial if there is any reason against it. Thus what is unacceptable to family physicians is unlikely to be done. There are also two practical advantages in this. Firstly, if a volunteer suffers from any condition or is receiving any treatment that makes participation in the trial undesirable, it is unlikely to be missed. Secondly, if the volunteer developed some symptoms which may or may not be connected with the trial, diagnosis and treatment could be difficult if the doctor did not know what the patient had taken. It seems of overwhelming importance that the medical practictioner whom a volunteer might see in an emergency should know about a trial. At the very least, it is a matter of courtesy. Of course courtesy (real courtesy, not etiquette), is the same as ethical conduct in small matters.

There are some other safeguards. People should not solicit volunteers among their subordinates but do it through a comparatively junior person to whom a refusal can be given without embarrassment and in the knowledge that refusals will not be reported. Those under the age of 14 should not be asked to volunteer, those under 18 only if the tests are quite harmless. If volunteers are below the age of legal majority, they should obtain their parents' permission, though it is usually enough if they report that a parent has approved. Service volunteers should be seen without their superiors. After they have been told what the trial involves, they should have the opportunity to withdraw, their superiors being told only that those not taking part were unsuitable for the trial. (Of course anyone unwilling is unsuitable.)

Inducements

There should never be a possibility that anyone might take part in a trial for the sake of inducements and against better judgement. It is difficult to avoid all inducements, for example patients may mistakenly expect more attention if they take part in a trial. For those conducting a trial and for those taking part in it, the main inducement should be to help medical research. This is not starry-eyed idealism. In a country where the first comprehensive blood transfusion service began and still continues entirely with voluntary blood donors it seems unwise to assume that volunteers in clinical trials should be paid. On the contrary, it is unethical to tempt anyone into volunteering, and only small awards can be justified.

To those working in the pharmaceutical industry there is a practical as well as an ethical argument against payment in cash or by gift vouchers, for these would be taxable as benefits obtained from the employers and related to the employer's business. My practice is to avoid all mention of awards but to give a good party to volunteers at the end of the experiment, to which spouses are also invited if the experiment was onerous.

Those unable to volunteer

Certain kinds of people cannot volunteer, especially mental patients and children under 14. Yet it may be necessary to do clinical trials on such people, especially for conditions that only afflict them. Psycho-therapeutic agents must be tested on those suffering from mental illness, vaccines or chemotherapy for measles or whooping cough must be studied in children. If those in the trial are likely to benefit from it, they need not volunteer and no problem arises. When something must be done for research but not in the patients' interest, then the best thing might be to take all known safeguards together. Approval should be obtained from the Committee on Safety of Drugs, the Management Committee of the Hospital, the parents or next of kin and, insofar as this is at all possible, the patients themselves. This, combined with the good sense of reputable investigators, should meet ethical requirements.

Those in prison are by definition also unable to make free decisions. In Britain experiments are never done on prisoners. The argument is that inducements by privileges, or by remission of sentence, or even by relief of boredom, are so powerful that they might make prisoners agree to experiments which they would not do otherwise. In the United States the first people to take new remedies are often prisoners, though the best prisons and most pharmaceutical companies insist on as much care as if the research director himself was an experimental subject. The argument in favour of this practice is that those who have offended against the laws of the community should have a chance to redeem themselves and that it is humane to give prisoners the opportunity of earning privileges or early release by a voluntary act of service. But not all prisoners can be given this opportunity, and the authorities must select those who can volunteer. This further limits the prisoners' freedom. The ethics of this have been carefully considered. (*Journal of the American Medical Association,* 1948). Yet, one cannot help wondering whether this is as good a safeguard as finding volunteers among those who developed the new substance and among the patients likely to benefit from it.

Relationships between doctors and volunteers

It has been suggested that a volunteer becomes a patient if he receives a pharmacologically active substance from a registered medical practitioner or if he develops any symptoms as a result of an experiment (Glaser, 1964). It seems reasonable to assume that a decision to volunteer may be influenced by the fact that the experimenter or one of the experimenters is a medical man, and it is inevitable that a doctor-patient relationship should be established by giving an active substance. This has not been tested before the courts or the General Medical Council, and it is to be hoped that it never will be. But it is well to remember that a moral responsibility exists. Anything that would offend medical ethics in relation to a patient would presumably be unacceptable in relation to experimental volunteers.

The duty to be effective

If patients or volunteers and medical or auxiliary staff spend their time and energy on a clinical trial, there is a moral duty that the trial should be run well. Most of the present symposium is concerned with the quality of clinical trials. But it should be stated firmly that quality is an ethical as much as a scientific responsibility (Pickering, 1949; Bean, 1959; Royal College of Physicians, 1967; Black, 1968). If it is unethical not to compare treatments, it must be unethical to fail because of bad design or sloppy execution. The skill of the experimenter is to combine the demands of medicine and science with those of ethics.

Conclusions

There can be no difficulty if common sense and common decency are always used. The rules are available and should be consulted. If in doubt, the answer is usually that which maintains the right relationship between a medical practitioner and his patients.

REFERENCES

BEAN, W. B. (1952). A testament of duty: some strictures on moral responsibility in clinical research. *J. Lab. clin. Med.* **39,** 3.

BEAN, W. B. (1959). Ethics of experimentation on human beings. In *Clinical Evaluation of New Drugs,* p. 76. Ed. Waife, S. O. & Shapiro, A. P. New York: Hoeber.

BLACK, D. A. K. (1968). *The Logic of Medicine,* p. 66. Edinburgh: Oliver & Boyd.

FOX, T. F. (1959). The ethics of clinical trials. In *Quantitative Methods in Human Pharmacology and Therapeutics,* p. 222. Ed. Lawrence, D. R. New York: Pergamon Press.

GLASER, E. M. (1964). Volunteers, controls, placebos, and questionnaires in clinical trials. In *Medical Surveys and Clinical Trials,* p. 115. Ed. Witts, L. J. London: Oxford University Press.

HILL, A. BRADFORD (1963). Medical ethics and controlled trials. *Brit. med. J.* **1,** 1043.

JOURNAL OF THE AMERICAN MEDICAL ASSOCIATION (1948). Ethics governing the service of prisoners as subjects in medical experiments. **136,** 457.

McCANCE, R. A. (1951). The practice of experimental medicine. *Proc. R. Soc. Med.* **44,** 189.

MEDICAL RESEARCH COUNCIL (1963). Responsibility in investigations on human subjects. *Annual Report,* 1962-3, H.M.S.O., reprinted in *Br. med. J.* (1964) **2,** 178.

PICKERING, G. W. (1949). The place of the experimental method in medicine. *Proc. R. Soc. Med.* **42,** 229.

PIUS XII (1952). Moral limits of medical research. Address to the first international congress on the histology of the nervous system. *Catholic Mind* (1953). **51,** 305.

ROYAL COLLEGE OF PHYSICIANS (1967). Supervision of the ethics of clinical investigations in institutions. *Br. med. J.* **3,** 429.

WOLSTENHOLME, G. E. W. & O'CONNOR, M. (1966). *Ciba Foundation Symposium on Ethics in Medical Progress.* London: Churchill.

WORLD MEDICAL ASSOCIATION (1964). Declaration of Helsinki. *Br. med. J.* **2,** 177.

WORLD HEALTH ORGANIZATION (1968). Principles for the clinical evaluation of drugs. *Tech. Rep. Ser. Wld Hlth Org.* No. 403.

LEGAL CONSIDERATIONS IN DRUG EVALUATION

D. R. CHAMBERS

During the course of the symposium different definitions of clinical trial have been given. The Medicines Act 1968, sec. 31 (1) states:

> In this Act 'clinical trial' means an investigation or series of investigations consisting of the administration of one or more medicinal products of a particular description—
> (a) by, or under the direction of, two or more doctors or dentists to one or more patients of his, or
> (b) by, or under the direction of, two or more doctors or dentists, each product being administered by, or under the direction of, one or other of those doctors or dentist to one or more patients of his,
> where (in any such case) there is evidence that medicinal products of that description have effects which may be beneficial to the patient or patients in question and the administration of the product or products is for the purpose of ascertaining whether, or to what extent, the product has, or the products have, those or any other effects, whether beneficial or harmful.

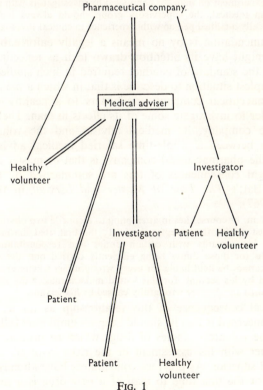

FIG. 1

Parties to clinical investigations and volunteer studies.

It is now recognised by statute that the administration of a drug may result in harmful effects. One legal consideration in clinical trials is, therefore, if harmful results do occur during a clinical trial, who is to pay? I know of no case in which an English court has been expressly concerned with this problem so that direct legal authority about the matter is unavailable. Nevertheless it is possible to examine some of the legal principles involved in both clinical trials and human volunteer studies.

The possible parties who might be concerned in a clinical trial or human volunteer study are set out in the figure. From this it can be seen that such investigations are possible without the direct intervention of a medically qualified person, in particular the medical adviser of the company concerned. The recommendations of the Royal College of Physicians on clinical trials (1967) have been referred to by earlier contributors. Here I would refer only to one of the recommendations which states:

> In non-medical institutions or wherever clinical investigation—that is, any form of experiment on man—is conducted by investigators with qualifications other than medical, the supervisory group should always include at least one medically qualified person with experience in clinical investigation.

This recommendation is by no means a legally enforceable rule, but any court might have its attention drawn to it as reflecting informed opinion on the standard of conduct required in such studies.

The simplest situation to describe is that in which a medical adviser of a pharmaceutical company administers to a healthy volunteer a drug in order to investigate some of its effects in man. There are three parties: the company, its medical adviser and the volunteer. The relationship between a whole-time salaried medical adviser and his employer, the pharmaceutical company, is that of master and servant and the legal consequences of this are summarised by the present author of Batt's *The Law of Master and Servant* in these words (Webber, 1967):

> The problem, of course, lies in attempting to reconcile two obvious principles which must receive the acceptance of all: the first, that the master having entrusted his servants with certain duties and responsibilities must be responsible for those duties being efficiently carried out; the second, that a master cannot be held liable for every wrongful act whenever and however committed by his servant, for this would make a master the insurer of the public against any damage wrongfully caused by his servant.

The practical consequence of this relationship as far as a medical adviser is concerned is that he should keep his employers fully informed about all the volunteer studies of drugs which he proposes to undertake, together with his assessment of the risks involved and that of any medical superior. As previous contributors have already observed, the giving for the first time to man of a new drug is a most critical step (e.g. Binns, Downie, Glaser). There are some differences of opinion which have been alluded to on the question of how much of a drug it is reasonably safe to give to man on the basis of the amount of relevant animal toxicity investigations which have been performed on it. This is one of the first matters which, I think, would concern a court should the matter be litigated.

Were a volunteer to threaten legal action because of injury arising during or from a drug given to him as a volunteer in a study, I think, he could try to claim first that he had never consented to accept the risks of the study or that the company through its medical adviser had been negligent in its conduct, or both. The comments of a high court judge who is also medically qualified (Ormrod, 1968), though directed more to the consent of volunteers to donate a kidney are, in my opinion, just as relevant to the present topic. He says:

> The field can be narrowed a good deal further by the law of trespass—that is, it is an actionable wrong to interfere bodily with another person without his consent in the absence of clear therapeutic indications. This raises a dilemma which has been the playground of jurists for centuries and which looks like becoming a medical nightmare in the twentieth century —'When is consent not consent?' The jurists have produced many learned but unsatisfactory answers; the doctors seem at present about to repeat the same sterile disputation. It is extremely difficult to produce any satisfactory abstract answer. Phrases such as 'real consent', 'informed consent', etc., merely raise new questions—what is meant by 'real', what is meant by 'informed'? But in practice and in the individual case it is not very difficult to decide whether someone has or has not effectively consented. Judges or juries manage to do it many times a year. If the consent has been obtained by trick the law will treat it as no consent; on the other hand, failure to provide all the relevant information will not necessarily invalidate it.

and also:

> Generally speaking, the law puts a heavy burden on the party who asserts that his apparent consent was not valid. In certain cases where one party is in a peculiarly weak position in relation to the other the law requires uberrima fides—that is, good faith and disclosure of all relevant facts. The relation of doctor and patient is one of these. Underlying the law's approach is the presumption that in general people over 21 are grown up and must take their own decisions. The law is not concerned with the motives or even the pressures which lead to their decision unless the latter are so severe as to overwhelm their minds.

The advice given in the recent W.H.O. technical report on principles for the clinical evaluation of drugs (1968) is also to the point and I quote.

4.1 Consent of subjects

> Subjects must usually be informed of the nature and the purpose of the trial and of the potential risks and benefits. A fair presentation of the major issues should be given, but not an excessively detailed and technical discussion, which might simply confuse the subject. A written record of the subject's consent is ordinarily desirable, although it need not contain an account of the full discussion required to acquaint the subject with the hazards and goals.

Previous authors have also observed that the first persons to be given a new drug are those fairly closely concerned with its development and so likely to be well acquainted with the risks of taking it. I am by no means convinced, however, that mere knowledge of a risk is on that account alone evidence of acceptance of that risk. The principle which appears to lie behind the maxim, 'volunti non fit injuria', requires both. I also think that the fact that the investigators who administer the drug and the volunteers who take it, are employees of the company who made it (indeed the first volunteer may be an investigator), raises problems based on the master and servant relationship mentioned earlier, in the field for instance of conditions of employment and the duties owed by and to fellow servants. The problems which could be so raised are too wide to be discussed further here, as so much would turn on the particular facts of any set of circumstances. Whatever the risks may be and however varied the possible circumstances from which injury could result from the investigations of drugs on volunteers, I think that companies can and ought to be insured against them. Certainly it is not reasonable to expect the medical adviser or his defence society to shoulder this burden, and my own enquiry with my own society has left me in no doubt how I stand in this regard. I would recommend that any of my colleagues who have problems of this sort take them up with their own society, as individual circumstances differ so widely.

On the question of negligence in drug studies the W.H.O. report states this:

4. 6 Compensation for injury

It is not possible under common law to absolve the investigator from liability for negligence; nor should he be so absolved. Liability for negligence remains a useful check on the incompetent or unscrupulous investigator. However, injuries or mishaps with medical consequences may occur during the course of research in which there is no question of negligence.

There has been a failure to consider the needs of human subjects who are injured in the course of an ethically irreproachable human experiment. There is need for some process, such as an insurance system, that will pay for medical care, where necessary, and provide appropriate compensation when research subjects sustain injury or death during investigation, regardless of possible negligence and without prejudice to liability. The cost of this protection should be considered part of the basic cost of the conduct of the clinical investigation.

What constitutes negligence is a matter to be decided from the facts of any particular case but any plaintiff alleging this must show that the person or persons whom he charges with negligence owed him a duty of care, that they have failed to maintain a reasonable standard of care and that as a consequence the plaintiff has suffered damage assessable in money terms.

In my opinion, a distinction has to be drawn between the drugs undergoing clinical trial and which have been 'approved'* for this purpose by the Committee on Safety of Drugs and drugs not so 'approved'. Unless the courts are to invoke a higher standard than that applied by those experts charged with the specific duty of deciding

* Although letters from the Committee seldom use the term 'approved', the Annual Report for 1967 uses the term 'approved' in its Appendix III, Submissions dealt with in 1967.

whether a drug should be submitted to clinical trials,** then approval by this Committee implies that the required standard of drug safety has been complied with.

This is always subject to the proviso that the ' approved ' drug has been administered in accordance with any conditions which may have been laid down by the Committee and that the company has made a full disclosure of the relevant facts to them. Similar reasoning applies to the use of an ' approved ' drug in a volunteer study. What to me is not quite clear is the position when a drug as yet for which there is no ' Dunlop approval ' is given to man and injury results. What would be the attitude of a court if a widow claimed damages for negligence based on the death of her previously perfectly healthy husband who collapsed and died seconds after the intravenous injection of an experimental compound? My feeling is that on some reasoning or other, possibly by invoking the doctrine of ' res ipsa loquitur ', i.e. ' the thing speaks for itself ', the court would find for the plaintiff. So far as I know this dire eventuality has never occurred, but I (no less than the W.H.O. expert committee) would like to be reassured that if it did, it should not be the volunteer's family who bears this load. Since delivering this paper I have heard that the A.B.P.I. has set up a committee to examine this problem of human experimentation and I look forward to its findings and recommendations with the keenest interest.

So far I have considered the company, the medical adviser and the volunteer. The patients in clinical trials are, however, no less volunteers and their consent to the study must be obtained and recorded in the manner noted above. Supposing such a patient alleges injury during a study, to whom would he look for recompense? Probably a patient could join as defendants the doctors treating him, the authorities of the hospital in which he was treated, the company whose drug it was and its medical adviser. A few words of comfort now for the hospital doctors:

> It is difficult to see how any outside body can do more than protect the doctor in his positive decisions and expose his negative decisions to criticism. The role of such lay persons can never be more than advisory. There are, of course, advantages in being able to discuss such difficult decisions with other people who may have different views or different sources of information, but the doctor cannot share the decision any more than the judge. This is, I think, clearly recognized in the recent report of the Committee of the Royal College of Physicians over which Sir Max Rosenheim presided, but, if I may respectfully say so, I have some difficulty in agreeing with the views of that committee that the ultimate responsibility for the proper conduct of clinical trials rests with the hospital or medical school authorities in whose premises such trials are conducted. It may be that a patient who has suffered damage in such a trial would be able to sue the hospital or medical school as employers of the doctors concerned, but the hospital would undoubtedly be entitled to look to those doctors to pay the resulting damages and costs. (Ormrod, 1968.)

** Ibid. Appendix I.

In practice hospital doctors and general practitioners are likely to find their interests safeguarded by their defence societies and by the existence of 'Dunlop approval', but as hospital management committees are possible parties to an action based on allegations of negligence arising from a clinical trial, it is hardly surprising that one should hear of objections to such studies being raised by such bodies, or of requests for indemnity from the risks arising from clinical trials.

In practice, as I observed earlier, neither clinical trials nor human volunteer studies have so far generated legal problems. The major credit for this must be attributed to those persons who have been concerned in such studies. It is clear to me, as it is to all participants in this symposium, that the precautions surrounding the administration of drugs in clinical trials are much more stringent than those commonly attending the administration of drugs to patients in the ordinary course of medical treatment. The standard required in investigating new drugs is getting higher, a fact which reflects great credit to all those concerned with the conduct of these investigations and the continued maintenance of such high standard will, I am certain, make the consideration of the legal aspects of clinical trials an academic exercise, until that is, the relevant provisions of the Medicines Act 1968 come into force.

REFERENCES

COMMITTEE ON SAFETY OF DRUGS (1968). Report for the year 1967. London: H.M. Stationery Office.
ORMROD, SIR ROGER (1968). Medical ethics. *Br. med. J.* **2**, 7.
ROYAL COLLEGE OF PHYSICIANS (1967). Report of the Committee on Supervision of Clinical Investigation. *Br. med. J.* **3**, 429.
WEBBER, G. J. (1967). *Batt's Law of Master and Servant*, 5th ed., p. 322. London: Pitman.
WORLD HEALTH ORGANISATION (1968). Principles for the clinical evaluation of drugs. *Wld Hlth Org. Tech. Rep. Ser.* No. 403.

INFORMATION RETRIEVAL

P. Wade

The term 'information science' is now passing from the reproach of jargon to the respectability of acceptance as a description of a discipline concerning itself with the investigation of the properties and behaviour of information, of the flow and use of information and of the methods, both manual and machine, used in storage, retrieval and dissemination of information.

Information retrieval therefore is one part only of a rapidly growing field of interest, but it is the part which most immediately affects the majority of scientists.

In itself information retrieval can mean many things. Asking the right question of the right man, or being associated with an information exchange group, is just as much information retrieval, as consulting a reference book, or an index; but in the main the term brings to mind first the use of published sources, reference books, abstracting services, and especially general indexes to periodical, and to a lesser extent, monographic publications.

It may be thought of as a continuous process of searching new publications, and new indexes to be made aware of the appearance of new work which may affect an existing interest of one's own, or even suggest an interest which one should perhaps take-up.

Equally it may have a more restricted and specific meaning, the search for past publication, of whatever date, bearing specifically on a particular piece of one's current work.

Whether one's concern is with the 'continuous' or 'up-dating search', or the 'retrospective' search (to use jargon terms for those two approaches) the one certainty is that the search 'for everything that has been published on . . .' is hopeless. Indeed perhaps there is some consolation in that fact otherwise the current bogy of the 'information explosion' may be too dismaying for many to contemplate. That bogy has been with us for longer than we generally realise, even if our ancestors did not add to their fears by coining a new horror term for it.

John Shaw Billings recognized the feeling of dismay at the increasing volume of publication in his paper *Our Medical Literature*, delivered at the International Congress of Medicine in London in 1881. He said ' The analogies between the mental and physical development of an individual, and of a nation or society have often been set forth . . . but there is one point where the analogy fails as regards the products of mental activity—and that is that as yet we have devised no process for getting rid of the exuviae . . . litera scripta manet . . .

Our literature is in fact something like the inheritance of the golden dustman, but with this important difference that when the children raked a few shells or bits of bone from the dustman's heap,—and after stringing them together and playing with them a little while, threw them back,—they did not thereby add to the bulk of the pile,—whereas our preparers of compilations and compendiums, big and little, acknowledged or not, are continually increasing the collection, and for the most part with material that has been characterized as " superlatively middling, the quintessential extract of mediocrity " . . . the really valuable part of the observations of the old masters has long ago become part of the common stock, and the results are to be found in every text book . . . Yet [a man] should know how to make [a bibliographical] search if only to enable him to direct others, and it is for this reason that a little acquaintance with bibliographical methods of work ought to be obtained by the student.'

Billings indeed practised what he preached. In the library of the Surgeon-General's Office (now the National Library of Medicine of the U.S.A.) he brought together a vast collection of publications; and in his creation of the Index-Catalogue of the Library of the Surgeon-General's Office, and of the Index Medicus he provided magnificent, universally applicable bibliographical tools for the retrieval of collected information. Since his day the number of general indexes, particularly to the periodical literature, has grown, and the methods of indexing have diversified. The conventional subject heading approach has its difficulties—the indexer and the searcher may have differing views on the allocation of subject terms or terms change their meanings over the years.

The difficulty of establishing an unequivocal starting point is recognized in the evolution of such an index as *Science Citation Index* which offers an unambiguous starting point, the personal name of a particular individual, known to the searcher as an authority in his particular field of interest. From that point it is assumed (and it appears, reasonably so) that works quoted by that particular individual, and works quoting him, are likely to be of value to the searcher; and the index is constructed to lead the searcher to those citations both backwards and forwards from his starting point—a personal name.

Other indexes have sought to develop methods for reducing the delay between appearance of a publication and the time at which reference to it appears in a general index by aiming at a reduction of the intellectual labour of conventional indexing and by seeking quicker methods of preparing the index for publication. From this came such forms as the KWIC indexes (Key Word in Context) with at least semi-mechanical selection of significant terms from the original publication, and mechanical manipulation of those terms to produce the index.

Alongside these and other forms of general indexes there has been a proliferation of devices aimed at giving a man an opportunity of keeping himself to some extent quickly aware of new publication in some field of general and continuing interest to him. To some extent the conventional abstracting journals, and the review journals might be so used. Again there was the worry (even though at times a somewhat exaggerated one) about the delay between publication of original matter and the time at which an abstract was published; and so there appeared collections of the contents-sheets of major current journals which a man could browse through quickly; a widely known example of course is *Current Contents.*

All those tools of information retrieval are in physical form conventional, printed (or near-printed) books, for use by an individual equipped with patience, a pencil and reasonable eyesight. A search made from them has come to be called a ' manual search ', presumably as distinguished from the ' machine search ' which generally implies the use of an information system based on a computer. Whether some other storage and retrieval systems, such for example as a feature-card index, which work on optical coincidence of holes punched in superimposed cards, should be regarded as 'manual' or ' machine ' searching systems could be a matter of taste in words, but the general tendency is to link ' machine search ' with the use of the computer in storage and retrieval of references.

One of the best known of these systems is MEDLARS—the Medical Literature Analysis and Retrieval System, developed by the National Library of Medicine of the U.S.A.

All journals covered by the system are scanned by indexers who allocate to each article index terms taken from the rigid vocabulary (MeSH; Medical Subject Headings) governing the system. The full indexing is in considerable depth with articles having as many as about ten indexing terms allocated.

Of course if indexing in that depth were reproduced in a conventional printed general index the result would be an index which would be too unwieldy, physically, for use in the ' manual search '. The Index Medicus is one product of the system but the entries there are restricted to the two or three indexing terms which the indexer indicated as reflecting the major interest of the article. Only the articles so tagged are recognized by that operation of the system operating the computer-driven phototypesetting for the monthly Index Medicus, and for the annual cumulative volumes.

For specific, individual, searches on a particular topic however the formulation of the ' search-statement ', the interrogation of the machine memory, can utilise the full depth of the indexing.

In the United Kingdom access to the resources of MEDLARS is available, generally through a librarian, in the U.K. MEDLARS Information Retrieval Service under the auspices of the National Lending Library ' Regional MEDLARS Liaison Officers ' are available to demonstrate the system and to arrange searches in Newcastle-upon-Tyne, London, Edinburgh and Manchester.

MEDLARS is of course one only of a number of machine retrieval systems in the course of development. All have virtues and limitations; all demand an approach both critical and understanding if the user is not to be (expensively) disappointed.

One of the most recently inaugurated services is the Drug Literature Computer Tape Service of Excerpta Medica Foundation, Amsterdam, which has been designed to meet requirements (from organizations with the equipment to handle IBM compatible tapes, and the resources to meet the annual subscription to the service) for ‘highly specific medical and chemical information on all experimental and marketed drugs and chemical compounds derived from the total international biomedical literature’. The service claims that it will be scanning more than 150,000 articles annually from approximately 3,500 biomedical journals.

All these searches of all varieties of index, and by all variety of means may be carried out to a greater or less extent either by the worker himself, or for him by a specialized information officer, or by a general librarian. There is much virtue in the worker himself making at least a preliminary search. His knowledge of his field will enable him to exercise more critical judgement in assessing what he wants to read, and leaving aside a vastly greater mass of material which he feels can be disregarded with little danger of anything vital being lost. Indeed that preliminary personal search may well suffice and save expenditure of time and money on the amassing by someone else of an enormous list of Billing's ‘ superlatively middling ’ literature.

It is indeed an essential part of information retrieval to exercise judgement on the time and effort which should be put into it in relation to any particular object. Its potential should never be overlooked, but there must be some degree, too, of resistance to the insidious temptation to go on looking for what some one else may have done without ever starting to try something oneself.

The outcome of a search will generally be a list of references, though of course some of these may be elaborated by the provision of annotations and abstracts to the point of becoming skeleton review articles. From the straightforward list of references the worker must decide which articles he wants to read; and getting those articles from local, national or international resources can be a trying task though librarians will generally do their utmost to alleviate it—particularly when given accurate and informative references. For the scientist in this country the problem has been greatly eased in recent years by the magnificent service of the National Lending Library for Science and Technology.

With the publication in his hand the worker comes to the crux of information retrieval; he must read the article.

INITIAL PREPARATION FOR CLINICAL TRIALS

J. A. L. GORRINGE

My paper starts in a sort of primeval wasteland where our primitive experimental drug is only just emerging from the steaming swamp of the pre-clinical laboratory work-up and discusses aspects that nobody knows very much about.

The title implies that even at this early embryonic stage in the gestation of a new drug one does have the distant daylight of ultimate delivery dimly in sight and one recognises that clinical trials of varying types in orderly sequence will be required if the drug is to develop normally through stages corresponding to organogenesis and subsequent intra-uterine growth.

For clinical trials you only need two things: investigators and patients. Even an experimental drug is not essential. You can equally well evaluate exercise against no exercise or brushing your teeth against not brushing your teeth. So I shall talk about investigators and patients. Did I call them earlier ' things that nobody knows very much about '? Well, I stand by that.

Patients and investigators have one thing in common; there are never enough of the right kind when you want them. It is natural when considering the choice of an investigator for a particular type of drug to think first of individuals who you know have previously carried out clinical trials of drugs of that class. This may be the main reason why many people tend to become specialists in a particular kind of clinical investigation. We can all think of men who are known mainly for their work in the evaluation of anti-hypertensive drugs, analgesics, oral contraceptives and anti-inflammatory drugs. No doubt there is satisfaction in knowing that you are an acknowledged expert but there is also frustration in knowing that you are type-cast. It is not therefore surprising that these specialist investigators not infrequently retire after a time into more academic pursuits and cease to be available for the conduct of clinical trials. From the point of view of the pharmaceutical company this tendency to specialise has the additional disadvantage that when clinical trials of one drug are finishing and trials of a different class of compound about to begin, one has to find a completely fresh set of investigators. Obviously one would not expect a rheumatologist to evaluate an anaesthetic but there is no fundamental reason why a cardiologist for example should not undertake clinical trials of diuretics, anti-hypertensive drugs, analgesics, anti-atheroma agents, fibrinolytic, anti-arrhythmic, anti-obesity and even bronchodilator drugs. Some will and the problem as a rule is to find out which.

When a man tells you he will gladly undertake the clinical trial you suggest to him it does not always follow that he will do so. There are, of course, unforeseen and unavoidable events that interfere: the individual accepts a new appointment, he becomes sick, he loses his registrar, he goes on a lecture tour to the United States but there is also the Macbeth syndrome. Lady Macbeth called her husband ' infirm of purpose ' because he lacked the resolution to carry through the project they had planned. We have all met investigators of whom the same may be said and it must always be our aim to identify the infirm of purpose and avoid them. It is wise to suspect the Macbeth syndrome when Binn's sign is present. Binn's sign consists in use by the investigator of the words ' leave it to me old boy '. Faced with Binn's sign one can sometimes confirm the diagnosis by the protocol test which consists in asking the investigator to sign the protocol to indicate his agreement with it and willingness to work as it specifies. Even with these diagnostic aids a few cases of the Macbeth syndrome are identified only retrospectively.

The man who says he will do a clinical trial and doesn't is especially irritating but let us not lose sight of the fact that probably 90 per cent of doctors would refuse outright. That is honest and one cannot criticise the individual doctor who does not wish to become involved in the demanding work of formal drug evaluation. One may legitimately complain, however, that *so many* do not wish to do so. Every doctor would say, if you asked him, that he has a right to expect the drugs he uses to have been thoroughly tested before they are made available to him. He is perfectly right. Everybody recognises that the job does have to be done. Why then do so many doctors think it should be done by somebody else?

Numerous reasons are given for declining to undertake a clinical trial, but very few people say bluntly that they are not interested. Even fewer admit that they have misgivings about their ability to handle the job. Yet I believe these two reasons, though rarely stated, are not infrequently the true ones. There are still many medical men including first class senior physicians who feel that their job is largely done when they have made a diagnosis. The houseman can take care of the treatment. I am perhaps exaggerating a little—but only a little. There really are members of our profession to whom therapeutics is a second-class branch of medicine. While this attitude is prevalent one must expect that only a small minority of doctors will undertake therapeutic trials.

If interest in and proper understanding of therapeutics is often lacking the blame must lie largely with the medical schools. I believe the subject is adequately taught in more medical schools today than it was when I was a student and one must hope that this trend will continue but teaching therapeutics in the narrow sense is not quite enough. As a one-time student of Professor, now Sir Derrick Dunlop, I was taught how to treat patients by probably the greatest teacher of the art in Britain at that time but I was a registrar before I was first required to think about the way in which different treatments can be scientifically compared. The basic techniques of drug evaluation, including even a little elementary statistics, are being taught nowadays in more medical schools than was once the case but still not enough. To a greater or less extent comparing one treatment with another is part of every doctor's job. Is it not reasonable to demand that his training shall include instruction in how best to do it?

Until medical schools can get it across to their students that the therapeutic revolution is not over and that its future progress will depend upon them, there will continue to be a chronic shortage of competent investigators.

The most essential qualification of an investigator is that he should have or have access to an appropriate number of suitable patients. I have already talked about some of the factors affecting the supply of investigators; the supply of patients is a totally different matter. It is governed by Lasagna's Law. I expect many of you are already familiar with Lasagna's Law. It can be represented graphically (Fig. 1) by a square wave, the periodicity of which is determined by the duration of a clinical trial. As soon as the trial begins the supply of suitable patients becomes one tenth of what it was said to be before the trial began. I have assumed that it returns to the pre-trial level as soon as the trial ends.

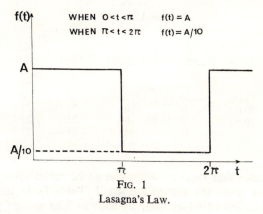

FIG. 1

Lasagna's Law.

What causes the curious disappearance of suitable patients as soon as we initiate a clinical trial? Usually **we** do. By ' we ' I mean medical advisers in the industry or anyone else who undertakes the detailed planning of a trial. In the interests of safety, ethical considerations and accepted standards of design, we stipulate patient selection criteria that exclude a high proportion of the available population. To insure safety we exclude those who are or may become pregnant, those in whom possible contra-indications exist to the use of experimental or control drugs, those who are receiving or have previously received treatment that might interfere with the effect of trial medication, those with a history of allergic phenomena, those with laboratory test results outside a specified range and often a host of other features that may be thought possibly to increase the hazards. Often we decide that it would be unethical to include certain categories of patients in case they should be allocated to placebo treatment. Certainly it would be unethical to include patients who are unwilling to take part.

Everyone who writes about the design of clinical trials contributes to the operation of Lasagna's Law by insisting upon certain design criteria such as precision of diagnosis, homogeneity of groups, comparability of groups and occasionally even matched pairs of patients.

Writing recently in Prescriber's Journal, Professor Graham Wilson (1968) covered all these points, and went on to say ' Elaborate statistics cannot validate a poorly designed or executed trial '. I agree with him of course but neither can elaborate statistics compensate for inadequate numbers of patients however well-designed and well-executed the trial may be. I do not dispute the desirability of Professor Wilson's design requirements and, when we are dealing with a very common disease entity, they may all be met in full. When dealing with less common conditions some compromises must be accepted. It is no use writing a perfect protocol for a trial that cannot be carried out.

TABLE I
Comparability of Groups

Drug	Dose	Males	Females	Total	Age (Mean)	Weight (Mean)
CI-572	25 mg	16	6	22	20·6	10 st. 5 lbs.
CI-572	50 mg	19	4	23	21·0	10 st. 6 lbs.
DF-118	60 mg	16	6	22	21·1	10 st. 6 lbs.
Placebo	—	18	5	23	21·3	11 st. 5 lbs.

Remember also that randomisation cannot be relied upon to provide comparability when the groups are small (Table I). In this table the random allocation of 90 medical students to four groups produced a substantial mis-match in weight. By luck the placebo group was the odd one and this didn't matter too much. Comparability of groups is by far the most important factor in determining the validity of a clinical trial and the easy way to achieve comparability is to use a lot of patients. This is why Lasagna's Law is such a serious bugbear.

At the very earliest stage of preparation for clinical trials it is as well to consider how many patients may be needed and how to get them. A statistician could talk for hours about estimating sample sizes but I'm not a statistician and I haven't got hours. I must assume that with appropriate statistical help you can reach a conclusion as to the minimal sample size that will make a proposed trial feasible. If the number of patients thought to be available is greatly in excess of this calculated minimal number, you can plan something approaching an ideal clinical trial and the next speaker will tell you how to do that.

I can only suggest a few things that you should *not* do when the adequacy of the numbers available is questionable.

First, don't ask for matched pairs. This wastes 50 per cent of a patient population due to pairing failure alone. That is one of the falacies of the reputedly economical sequential trial. Another is that a matched pair who respond equally to the drugs being compared are also wasted.

Secondly, if you have to choose between homogeneity and comparability, don't compromise with comparability. Relax your acceptance criteria and resort to stratified randomisation. You may, for example, accept out-patients as well as in-patients, provided that you allocate the same number of each to each group. In the same way, if specifying ' classical rheumatoid arthritis ' according to A.R.A. criteria provides too few patients, you may have to include the ' definite ' and even the ' probable ' categories as well. This type of compromise contains a hidden bonus: the less diagnostically definite cases of disease usually include those of recent onset who may be more responsive to treatment. This improves the sensitivity of the experiment.

Thirdly, don't divide your patients into more groups than is absolutely necessary. When you are evaluating an analgesic most of the pundits will tell you that you must have a morphine group *and* a placebo group. If you have only 50 or 60 patients available you had better ignore the pundits and compare your drug with morphine *or* placebo but not both.

Fourthly, if formal patient consent is to be sought, don't make it harder than necessary for the investigator to get it. The Baltimore group found that the great majority of patients agreed to participate in an analgesic trial involving post-operative pain if they were asked pre-operatively. If asked post-operatively when pain was actually present, an equal majority declined. Obviously an ethical problem arises here but it can usually be met by an escape clause permitting the use of other drugs if experimental medication is not rapidly effective.

Fifthly, don't insist upon the exclusion of certain categories of patients unless it is really essential. If a drug causes damage to the gastro-intestinal mucosa of experimental animals it would seem at first sight mandatory to exclude patients with a history of peptic ulceration but the argument loses much of its validity if the alternative treatments for the patient's condition are aspirin, phenylbutazone, indomethacin and corticosteroids. Even when animal studies suggest possible teratogenicity, it may still be quite proper to include married women of child-bearing age provided that they are taking oral contraceptives. One of our investigators used to send young women whom he wished to include in a clinical trial to see his wife who ran the family planning clinic.

Much more could be said about investigators and patients but I will conclude by re-emphasising that they are the essential components of clinical investigation; there are rarely enough of either but the investigator usually brings his patients with him. So when you have selected your investigator, do try not to exclude nine-tenths of his patients by prohibitively strict selection criteria and try to design your trial so as to make the most economical use of them.

REFERENCE

WILSON, G. M. (1968). Some notes on the interpretation of therapeutic trials *Prescribers' J.* **8**, 95.

PRELIMINARY DESIGN—THE IDEAL CLINICAL TRIAL

D. M. BURLEY

The ideal clinical trial has probably never been performed, or if it has, it has not been brought to my notice. In fact, the suggestion has been made that it is linked with the concept of the ideal drug and the ideal patient, both of which also seem to elude one. Nevertheless, it is useful to consider the stages of a trial in their ideal form so that one can travel from stage to stage more or less smoothly and predictably. Problems will then be thrown up which will always be solved, and we can leave the authors of other chapters to show that this is not always so easy.

There are various types of clinical trial that can be planned but I shall concentrate very largely on the controlled trial as it forms the centrepiece of drug evaluation techniques as we know them today. Whatever the type of trial the emphasis is on the word *planned*. There is no place for the unplanned experiment in clinical medicine—' just give these tablets to a few patients at random and see if they have any effect '—any more than there is a place for an unplanned experiment in the laboratory. Unplanned events may occur in the course of a planned experiment, however, and the quality of an investigator can often be judged by the diligence with which he searches for the cause and the use he makes of them. Serendipity plays a big part in the discovery of drug action and can be defined as ' the faculty of making happy and unexpected discoveries by accident '.

Pilot studies

These form a very useful and I believe essential part of most drug investigation. They are usually carried out as the first tentative administration of a drug to patients, immediately following human pharmacological studies in volunteers. Their purpose is to try and answer a few important questions which will then enable one to standardise the basic design of the subsequent controlled study. Such questions as, the dosage or dosage range, the optimum time and frequency of administration, likely complaints and side effects are best answered before the controlled study starts to avoid wastage of time, effort and sacrifice of patient material. The aim is to reduce the likelihood of the formal trial suffering from faulty administrative details or from something unsuspected, but avoidable, cropping up. A good example is provided by early pilot studies with the anti-inflammatory agent indomethicin, where an initially high dosage caused a high incidence of side effects in rheumatic subjects. A lowered dosage reduced these, but with retention of the desired anti-inflammatory effect.

The controlled clinical trial

At the centre of clinical drug research is the controlled study and its design is as fundamental as the three R's of the educational system. In fact its principal components are what I call the three P's—the Plotters, the Plot and the Prize. Not that I think clinical trials have any connection with burglary but because I find the simile convenient. I will first present the Plotters.

The Plotters: The Consultant
The Registrar
The Pharmaceutical Medical Adviser
The Pharmacist
The Statistician
The Ward-Sister

The Consultant is the ' grey eminence ' who is responsible for approving the whole plot (plan) and who can take into account all the relevant considerations with regard to his patients and staff.

The Registrar represents all the subordinates who so often are responsible for carrying out the day to day administration of the trial and make the records.

The Pharmaceutical Medical Adviser is the one who comes to the table with what may best be termed the pedigree of the drug; those who sired it, who nurtured it, who is backing it and what awards it has already won. I do not intend to elaborate the simile further. In addition to this he must be able to provide important information with regard to toxicity and what special laboratory tests will be needed to evaluate it. He must be able to offer facilities for the printing of protocols and proformae, the manufacturing of tablets in identical form, amateur or even professional statistical advice and must be prepared as a last resort even to help write the paper.

The Pharmacist is a collective noun which includes the man responsible in the Pharmaceutical Company for ensuring that the tablets or capsules are prepared adequately in identical form, or whatever is required, and also the Hospital Pharmacist who will have charge of the drug when it reaches the hospital and may well be responsible for issuing the tablets to the correct patients according to a randomisation scheme.

The Statistician is the enthusiast who has slide rules at his finger tips and tables of ' t ' and ' chi-square ' under his arm. Everybody recognises his value after the trial has taken place, but many people pay lip service to the importance of his presence among the plotters. To explain why the advice of a statistician is required at an early stage it is necessary to bear in mind that clinical trials have two important objectives.

I. To avoid accepting a drug that is useless (Type I error of clinical trials).

II. To avoid rejecting a drug which is of value (Type II error of clinical trials).

It is usual to pay great attention to the first of these objectives and this is perhaps one of the reasons why controlled clinical studies give a rather low proportion of positive results as compared with uncontrolled studies. A number of workers during the past have analysed results of groups of controlled and uncontrolled studies on a particular drug and have pointed out the low incidence of favourable results in the former. They deduce from this, to my mind often wrongly, that the controlled trials are a more accurate and reliable guide, but this is not necessarily so. It assumes at the outset that the controlled studies were done properly; whereas so often they are not and are weighted heavily in favour of giving what Bradford Hill has termed a 'non-proven' result. If one reduces to a low level the probability of rejecting the null hypothesis, (that hypothesis which presupposes that there is no difference between treatments under test), the greater the chance of rejecting a drug which is of value. The connecting link between the Type I and Type II considerations is in most cases 'numbers', and the statistician will tell you at what level of significance to set your objectives and how many patients will be required to minimise both Type I and Type II errors of clinical trials.

Having made a plea for the statistician I will now mention the Ward Sister who is also usually left out of the team. Her assistance is going to be invaluable to ensure that the drugs are administered to the patients as indicated in the protocols and she may also do a number of other very important jobs like making sure the doctors write up the findings properly and that the records do not get lost. Being a trained observer with special opportunities for studying the patient 'off-guard', she may also provide valuable information in respect of therapeutic action and toxicity.

Although I have presented the first team it is important to call in other specialists for advice on important jobs and here I am particularly thinking of the doctor in charge of the laboratory. As a matter of courtesy it is best not to drop on him a work load of scores of extra tests per week without warning. But, in addition he can often give advice of real value as to what tests are relevant, to say nothing of their normal values.

The Plot

Figure 1 gives a bird's eye view of the flow chart which has to be constructed so that each phase of the ideal clinical trial can be properly carried out. Each phase consists of a main function and a subsidiary consideration, and for convenience it will be analysed phase by phase. The importance of having a plan cannot be over-emphasised because it enables the participants to think logically about what they are doing and if nothing else a clinical trial must be a logically planned clinical

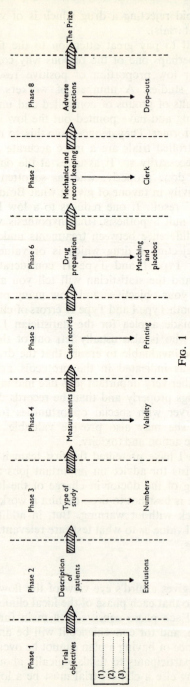

FIG. 1

experiment or investigation. Each member of the team will have responsibilities which can be allocated for each phase of the plot, although from time to time it may be necessary to modify some of the items to take account of the inevitable unexpected happenings which can wreck the progress of any trial if it is conducted in an atmosphere of vague hope. In our ideal clinical trial these possible mishaps will not occur and are, in any event, dealt with adequately in other chapters.

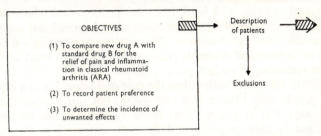

FIG. 2

Phase 1. The first decisions which have to be made concern the objectives (Fig. 2). In other words what questions are we going to try and answer as a result of our clinical trial? At the same time we should also be deciding whether these questions are in fact worth answering and whether we are justified in mounting a clinical trial to do so. It is part of our ethical concern for the prospective patients who will take part in the study. Generally speaking when one is treating disease groups, a new treatment or regime will be compared with what is regarded as the best of the old ones. If the old treatment is very effective then we shall need to have extremely good evidence from experimental and human pharmacological studies that the new regime will prove even better. On the other hand if previous treatments are poorly effective then we need less justification for trying something new and promising.

When comparing drugs for the relief of symptoms such as headache, pain and sleeplessness, our problem usually is to overcome the placebo effect of almost any regime, and the fact that the patients themselves will be aware that they are taking part in a study which involves potentially new remedies. Hence a group of patients on a placebo, or at least a period when all patients receive placebo treatment, may be an essential part of the investigation to get an idea of the extent of placebo reactions during the course of a trial. It is obviously not so necessary to ensure that the patient is getting the best of previously available remedies and, in any event, there could easily be very many of these with equal claims.

In Figure 2 three objectives are set out as an example. Under the first objective standard drug B is referred to. This could be one of a number of drugs for the condition under consideration, and in the standard treatment for rheumatoid arthritis simple analgesics such as aspirin and paracetamol, stronger antirheumatic agents such as phenylbutazone, its derivatives, and indomethacin, and specific anti-inflammatory agents such as the corticosteroids are included. All may be appropriate comparative drugs according to the nature and stage of the patients' disease. It is highly advisable also to define fairly precisely the disease which one is treating. So many cases are labelled rheumatoid arthritis with inadequate justification, and where possible one should seek a definition which bears some international acceptance and, in this case, the American Rheumatism Association's definition (1959) of definite and probable rheumatoid arthritis is most useful.

The recording of patient preference, particularly in trials involving the relief of symptoms rather than the cure of disease, is often essential. Some people may believe that one should not listen to anything the patient says, but in general what matters is whether the patient feels better and is able to perform daily tasks more efficiently and less uncomfortably. How these preferences are scored and charted can be considered under another heading

The determination of unwanted drug effects should be part and parcel of all drug trials and such effects are usually divided into side effects and toxic effects. Side effects are usually considered to be those effects which are inherent in the drug's pharmacological activity and which can often be predicted before the trial starts. They may be related merely to overdose, but sometimes they are unavoidable at therapeutic dosage. For example an overdosage of a short acting barbiturate may produce a hangover as well as a good night's sleep, but a diarrhoea producing dose of colchicine may be necessary to obtain the best relief in acute gout. Toxic effects are often unexpected and may consist of simple problems such as febrile reactions or transient rashes, to much more serious iatrogenic diseases such as drug induced retinopathy and agranulocytosis. Hence to achieve one's objective there is hardly a body system that should not be examined at intervals throughout any ideally performed clinical trial. Much discussion may be necessary before the correct balance is struck between what is necessary examination to protect the patient from untoward drug action and what is practicable in terms of doctor, nurse and laboratory capability.

Many other objectives may be built into the initial trial plans such as estimations of patient co-operation by pill returns, or urine tests for the presence of a drug. Also various social or psychological assessments can be brought in to determine the effect of the trial and the drugs on the patient's daily life, to say nothing of his preferences for different coloured capsules or tablets. However, it is usually as well to keep one's objectives to a manageable number like three or four, otherwise in its very complexity will lie the seeds of the trial's failure.

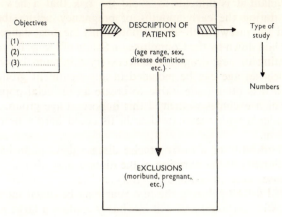

FIG. 3

Phase 2. Having set out the objectives of the trial the patient population must now be described precisely (Fig. 3) and suitable headings
will include the following topics :

1. Age range,
2. Sex,
3. Disease description,
4. Duration of the disease,
5. The status of a particular parameter of measurement,
6. Previous therapy,
7. Current therapy,
8. Source of patients.

For various reasons it may be necessary to exclude patients below
the age of 20 or above the age of 70 in certain trials. In the first
place the nature of the illness may be different at the extremes of age,
and above the age of 70 the liability of the patient to suffer from or
succumb to other illness not under investigation becomes increasingly
great. Children often need special consideration both in the management
of their condition and with regard to ethical problems and the need for
parental consent.

Obviously a disease which affects both sexes should have male and
female representatives when it is being studied, but the sex incidence
may be quite different as may the severity of the disease. For instance
in ankylosing spondylitis eight times as many males suffer from the
condition as females and the disease tends to run a milder course in
women. This might provide a reason for studying a regime of treatment on males and females separately. A further consideration which
has come into prominence since the teratogenic effects of thalidomide
were discovered in 1961 is the potential danger of new drugs to women
during their child bearing years. Apart from excluding women known

5

to be pregnant it is difficult to avoid the risk that a new drug will be taken during the early months of pregnancy before the state is recognised and just when the drug is potentially the most dangerous. The standards laid down by the Committee on Safety of Drugs for pharmacological testing of new drugs are a necessary minimum before women of child bearing age can be included in any treatment group. On the other hand it is often undesirable to create an artificial population of patients which excludes women of this important age group. A clinical trial in patients with rheumatoid arthritis could hardly be conducted without them.

The desirability of a fairly precise disease description has already been mentioned but the duration of the disease may also be important. Some diseases need to become 'established' to be regarded as typical. Rheumatoid arthritis during the first year may be much more difficult to classify with certainty and will inevitably contain a large number of cases with negative serology. Also response to treatment may be different. For this reason the Empire Rheumatism Council (1960, 1961) excluded 'first year cases' from the Gold Trial conducted in 1958.

When considering parameters of measurement it may be necessary to define the activity of the disease so as to avoid 'quiescent cases' or 'burnt out cases'. This is particularly necessary again when one considers rheumatoid arthritis and rather imprecise parameters such as the erythrocyte sedimentation rate (e.s.r.) may have to serve as an indication of disease activity. In trials involving hypotensive drugs certain limits may have to be set for diastolic or systolic blood pressure readings.

Previous therapy may have modified the course of a disease and present therapy may prejudice the evaluation of something new. To overcome these problems it may be necessary to have a 'run in period' before the trial proper begins. The length of this run in period will vary with the disease under investigation but if some previous treatments are stopped it may be some time before a 'steady state' is reached. Additional drug therapy may be used as an indicator of disease severity and in trials in rheumatic diseases the quantity of aspirin tablets taken by the patient is often used as a parameter to evaluate the effectiveness of a trial regime. That this procedure is fraught with dangers has been shown by Boardman and Hart (1967).

It is not often that the source of the patients is considered at all, and if I suggested that a sample of patients with rheumatoid arthritis should be taken from a gynaecological clinic it would be regarded as laughable. Nevertheless the mere fact that patients in a trial have been selected from a hospital population may mean that the sample is biased and not a true reflection of the disease picture. In fact apart from the patients all being women, rheumatoid arthritics selected through a gynaecological clinic might well be more representative of the true population than those attending a rheumatic unit.

The corollary to the description of the patient is the list of exclusions. Already the exclusion of pregnant patients has been mentioned, but it is also usual to define certain other groups who by reason of the severity of their illness or the presence of other pathology are unsuitable for inclusion in a clinical study.

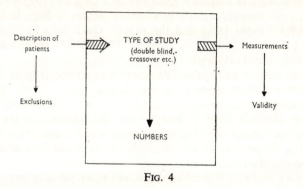

FIG. 4

Phase 3. The type of study may be defined broadly in terms of the mechanism: such as uncontrolled trials or controlled trials. On the other hand it may be described as a stage in the evaluation of a drug by such terms as pilot trial, definitive trial, promotional trial. We are concerned here with a controlled definitive study to answer precisely formulated questions, and we have to decide between such designs as (1) matched pair trial, (2) cross-over trial, (3) comparative group trial and (4) a combination of these.

The advantages and disadvantages of these designs has been well described by Maxwell (1968a). Because of the difficulty in matching pairs of rheumatoid arthritics our present trial would lend itself better to a cross-over type of study or if the numbers were sufficiently large, to a comparative group trial.

Hence the corollary to making a decision concerning the type of study is a consideration of the numbers of patients likely to be admitted to a trial. For group studies 25 to 50 patients may well be needed in each group, which could be beyond the reach of a single unit. Tables have been constructed by Clark and Downie (1966) and Maxwell (1968b) which give guidance concerning the number of patients required in comparative trials to obtain results at an approriate level of significance, minimising both Type I and Type II errors. In our particular trial as we cannot guarantee obtaining sufficient numbers of patients in a reasonable time we decided on a cross-over study which was in any event necessary if one was to record patient preferences, (objective 2).

Another method of obtaining a fairly large number of patients for a comparative group study is to involve several centres in what is known as a Multicentre Trial. These, however, carry their own particular problems and one of the most difficult is to ensure that the physicians responsible in each centre are agreed on the plan of the trial and that their individual understanding of that plan is the same. Good joint planning meetings are essential and a good central organiser such as a physician/statistician can go a long way towards making such trials run smoothly. Early multicentre studies of drugs in tuberculosis (M.R.C. 1948; 1950) and the E.R.C. Gold Trial in rheumatoid arthritis (Empire Rheumatism Council, 1960; 1961) are examples of where things went fairly well.

A good deal of mileage has been written on various types of blind study and the most popular is the double blind variety whereby different drugs, (with or without a placebo), are administered to the patient in identical form so that neither the patient nor the doctor recording the various observations is aware which preparation is being taken. The purpose of this is twofold: (1) to avoid bias and (2) to neutralise placebo effects.

The fact that this type of trial receives more plaudits from official and semi-official publications is no automatic guarantee of authenticity or validity. A double blind study requires thought and planning and this in itself is a good thing, but in many instances such a study is unnecessary or inappropriate. For example it may be possible to make comparisons directly with some standard response, such as haemoglobin rise following adequate treatment of iron deficiency anaemia (Swan and Jowett, 1959). In fact to get an instrument to produce the data by which drug response is to be judged is in itself a way of avoiding bias. Also it may be impossible to obtain drugs in identical form as for example when comparing a tablet regime with an injection regime. There are ways of overcoming this by the use of appropriate dummies, but so often the effort involved to preserve blindness is in itself prejudicial to the trial.

Finally one might mention triple and quadruple blind trials just to dispose of the notion that they describe trials of three or four drugs in identical form. In fact a triple blind trial jokingly refers to a situation where the Pharmacist who issues the drugs does not know what they are and in the quadruple blind trial the Statistician receives the data in randomised form so that he does not know which set of figures refers to which patient!

In rheumatic disease it is usually easy to put up and administer drugs in identical form and hence the double blind technique is appropriate and almost essential because so many of our observations are going to be subjective. Having decided upon this we consult with the Statistician who will help us to determine the degree of significance we might look for to avoid Type I and Type II errors and hence determine the number of patients to be admitted to our crossover trial. We will include a placebo regime to obtain an estimate of the sensitivity of the trial, for if no significant difference can be demonstrated between the present standard drug regime and the placebo, it will be hard to draw much in the way of conclusions as between the new regime and the standard regime.

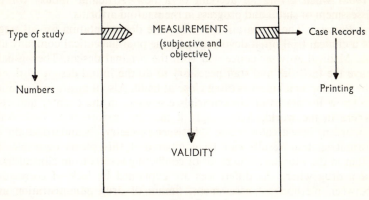

FIG. 5

Phase 4. The problem of parameters of measurement was discussed at length at a symposium on measurement in therapeutic assessment in 1965 (R.S.M. 1966) and the most important corollary to devising any new method is to carry out extensive investigations to assess the validity of the measurement in question in measuring what it is supposed to measure, and also whether that measurement is a useful guide to the progress and status of the patient's disease. One often feels that the ingeniousness of the method of obtaining the measurement or parameter bears an inverse relation to its value for the assessment of clinical status.

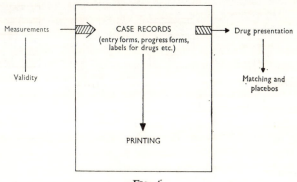

FIG. 6

In assessing methods of measurement it is its reproduceability, not only within observers, but also *between* observers, that is important.

So often the doctor making the measurements when a trial starts is not the one who is making the measurements at the end and therefore a considerable ' between observer ' difference in recording will be highly prejudicial. These problems were recently discussed by Ritchie *et al.* (1968) when giving an account of a new 'Articular Index' for the assessment of status and progress in rheumatoid arthritis.

Phase 5. The preparation of adequate documentation for all stages of a clinical trial often devolves upon the pharmaceutical company and the Medical Adviser concerned with the original design. They usually have the facilities and staff necessary to do the initial design work and the printing machinery is often close at hand. Also they are in a position to know the status of clinical trials elsewhere in the country and elsewhere in the world. Accordingly it may be important to have some ' between investigator ' and ' between country ' standardisation of format so that results can be compared if this seems desirable. So often in the literature one reads of conflicting results from clinical trials of a drug where the differences are explained by lack of correlation between methods of assessment, timing of drug administration and such like.

ENTRY FORM

PRETREATMENT RESULTS

NAME: ....   STUDY NUMBER: ....

Previous drugs: S   P   I   Et.   S   C   Others

X-RAY   Date   [   ]

Date sent   [   ]

EYES Ophthalmologists report   Normal [   ]   Other ....

Ward visual acuity R $\frac{6}{}$ L $\frac{6}{}$ ....

RENAL   **ELECTROLYTES**

Urine protein   [   ]   Calcium   [   ] mEq

Casts   [   ]   Sodium   [   ] mEq

Blood urea   [   ] mg%   Potassium   [   ] mEq

Creatinine clearance   [   ] ml/min   Chloride   [   ] mEq

BLOOD   **LIVER**

W.B.C.   [   ] /cu mm

Differential: Neut. [   ] % Lymph. [   ] % Eos [   ] %   S.G.P.T. [   ] Units

Baso. [   ] % Mono. [   ] %   Bilirubin [   ] mg%

Other

THERAPY   Weight   [   ] kg

Rifampicin [   ] mg   Ethambutol [   ] mg   Capreomycin [   ] mg

Date treatment started   [   ]

Signature ....

FIG. 7

THERAPY FOLLOW-UP

Patient	Week No.	Date	Normal Vision	Urea mg%	Sputum (if available) Smear	Culture	SGPT Units	Bilirubin mg%	Calcium mEq	Potassium mEq	W.B.C.	Differential N	L	E	B	M	Urine Prot.	Casts	TOXICITY AND REMARKS
Name:	2		Yes / No																Date treatment started ....
Study No:	4		Yes / No																
	6		Yes / No																
	8		Yes / No																Signature...............
Name:	10		Yes / No																
Study No:	12		Yes / No																
	14		Yes / No																
	16		Yes / No																Signature...............
Patient	Week No.	Date	Normal Vision	Urea mg%	Smear	Culture Sputum (if available)	SGPT Units	Bilirubin mg%	Calcium mEq	Potassium mEq	W.B.C.	N L E B M Differential					Prot. Casts Urine		TOXICITY AND REMARKS

FIG. 8

Entry Forms and Progress Forms for the patients in the trial should be precisely constructed and where possible the answers should be able to be recorded with the minimum of labour and maximum of clarity; the former will increase the chance of the form being filled in and the latter the ability of the statistician to interpret the answer. ' Yes—No ' boxes may be used for appropriate checking and other boxes for filling in results of specified tests. In follow up forms it is as well to specify the precise intervals at which various assessments and tests are to be repeated.

Two examples are shown of an Entry Form (Fig. 7) and Follow Up Form (Fig. 8), used in a trial of antituberculous agents where some of these principles are observed. Note on the Follow Up Form the hatching which indicates that certain repeat tests are not required at the 2, 6, 10 and 14 week intervals. It is also best to have some method of duplicating the records. Carbons are messy, but a flimsy made of NCR paper (No Carbon Required) can be torn off in strips if necessary as the results come in. Hence one has a complete durable record and a flimsy which can be despatched elsewhere for interim analysis and storage. If for some reason a record is destroyed the existence of a duplicate will prevent a set of results being lost to the analysis.

Finally time must be allowed for the printing of the various documents which may be considerable if the work has to be performed by a private printing company.

Phase 6. The next phase in the trial plan is to prepare the drugs for administration and in the case of the present study both standard drug and placebo are to be administered on the double blind principle, hence the subsidiary requirement in this phase will be the need for

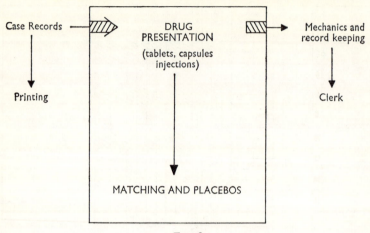

FIG. 9

identicality (Fig. 9). Considerable time, trouble and effort is needed to produce an acceptable match so that the identity of the drugs and the placebo cannot easily be detected by patient or doctor. Criteria have been laid down by Joyce (1968) for the production of matching drugs and are shown in Figure 10. It may appear that taken as a whole the criteria are rather stringent and virtually impossible to achieve, but for the ideal trial the attempt must be made for to fall short increases the risk of the treatments being correctly identified before the code is broken.

MINIMAL SPECIFICATION TO MANUFACTURERS OF CAPSULES OR TABLETS TO BE USED IN A COMPARATIVE TRIAL

1. To match perfectly* for:
   (a) Shape
   (b) Size
   (c) *Surface* colour
   (d) *Surface* texture
   (e) Weight

2. To match as closely as possible for:
   (a) Taste on licking
   (b) Taste on chewing
   (c) *Internal* colour
   (d) *Internal* texture
   (e) Smell
   (f) Specific gravity

3. To bear no external distinguishing signs, and to be put up in containers free of identifying marks. The containers for each treatment should be packed in separate boxes labelled with the identity of their contents.

   * Samples must be indistinguishable to a panel of four judges.

FIG. 10

Having mentioned the code it is also convenient here to draw attention to need for randomisation of drug administration. This will already have been considered when the trial design was discussed with the statistician in Phase 3. If two substances, A and B, are to be administered then there are only two possible orders that they can be given— namely AB and BA. If there are three agents A, B and C there are six possible orders: ABC, ACB, BAC, BCA, CAB and CBA.

The allocation of these various treatment sequences to the individual patients as they are admitted to the trial should be done by using some arbitrary device such as a table of random numbers. Hill (1967) gives such tables in his book *Principles of Medical Statistics* with instructions on how to use them.

Problems will arise during drug administration if it is necessary to allow for an increase in dosage for patients not responding. It is relatively easy to overcome this in single blind trials without the patient's knowledge by the use of dummy tablets for which the active drug is gradually substituted. Hence a patient may receive six identical tablets throughout all phases of the trial of which any number from nought to five may be dummies. In fact all six can be dummies during the placebo phase of administration. If the doctor is to remain ' blind ' as well then it will be necessary for the doctor making the observations on the patient to make some comment such as ' satisfactory response ' or ' inadequate response ' and a second doctor will act on these comments to alter the drug dosage up to some agreed maximum. It will usually be possible to avoid this sort of arrangement in trials of anti-rheumatic drugs, but in the treatment of a condition such as hypertension where the dose of a drug producing a desired response will vary from patient to patient such an arrangement may be mandatory.

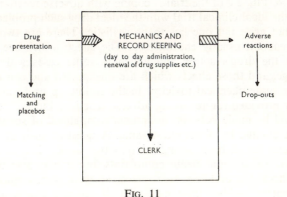

FIG. 11

Phase 7. At Phase 7 the trial can at last begin and the problem becomes one of mechanics and record keeping with its corollary the need for an efficient clerk or ' dogsbody '. Correct record forms have to be produced as the patients are entered in the trial and appear for follow up. The drugs must not run out, so the pharmacist must have an intermediate who can ensure that further supplies are obtained as required from the pharmaceutical company. As they are completed the forms must be stored away safely and any duplicates sent off to the statistician or other presiding doctor, as appropriate. In some trials it may be necessary to post letters or cards to remind out-patients that follow up visits are due and in the case of defaulters even a visit to the home may be required. The job of clerking the trial often devolves on the Ward Sister who has an office and a telephone, but ideally it should be somebody who does not regularly go off duty during crucial periods of the day. It is usually the house doctor, therefore, who is ' blooded ' in the routine of clinical trials by taking on this arduous task.

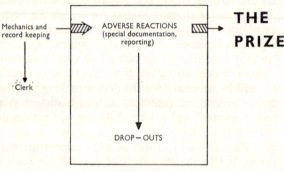

Fig. 12

Phase 8. Phase 8 of the trial is coping with adverse reactions as they arise. In the ideal clinical trial with the ideal drug such problems would perhaps not arise but one has to be realistic. There are two types of adverse reaction usually encountered. The effects which are part and parcel of the drug's action and which in some cases will represent overdosage, and those effects which are unexpected and can be due to allergy or some chemical toxicity. In the follow up proforma a space is usually provided for recording adverse reactions but a clear distinction should be made between symptoms complained of spontaneously and those elicited by direct questioning. A question such as ' how has your general health been during the past two weeks ' is a good way of finding out about spontaneous complaints, but it may also be best to have a check list of likely side effects as well, to ask about if one is deliberately seeking their incidence. If adverse effects are severe the patient may have to be withdrawn from the trial, alternatively such effects may be a reason for defaulting from follow up. If patients do ' drop out ' in this way every effort must be made to find the reason. It is important to know the incidence of adverse reactions in the evaluation of a drug and because a patient in a trial has stopped attending it must not be assumed that he is cured or has left the district.

The 'drop outs' from the trial will have to be included in the eventual analysis, unless it can be shown that their treatment has been incomplete for reasons unconnected with the progress of their disease and the therapy. In such circumstances it may be permissible to substitute another patient for the drop-out case.

Special documentation is desirable for the recording of adverse reactions and an example of such a form is shown in Figure 13, and is used by the Federal Drugs Administration of America. It contains the sort of detail that is necessary for recording adverse effects encountered during the course of a clinical trial.

As time passes our trial gradually comes towards completion and to our surprise it has not taken longer to complete than we had first calculated in the days of its conception. However, post-maturity is the rule and most trials take many months longer to complete than the original estimate. Patients whom one was seeing in scores before a trial starts have an annoying habit of disappearing the moment the bell rings. With the passage of time interest wanes and one wonders whether the blessed trial is ever going to end. However, the day dawns when one can reach for *The Prize*. It is a small parcel of legibly and correctly filled in documents recording the progress of all the patients throughout the course of the trial, with measurements and assessments both objective and subjective. It can be passed on with confidence to the statistician in the sure knowledge that a successful paper is about to be born.

General practitioner trials

General practitioner trials are sometimes frowned upon, but so much of the medical relief of annoying symptomatology takes place entirely outside hospital, and can only be evaluated practically in the context of general practice. Once again the difficulty in agreeing on the precise definition of the patients to be included in the trial is a major problem, (fibrositis and sciatica mean different things to different doctors). Several groups of practitioners have however made a great success of carrying out scientific general practitioner trials and provided it is done as a set piece and not something that is attempted as and when one has time while wading through a waiting room full of people, valuable information can be obtained about the use of analgesics, hypnotics, appetite suppressants, etc.

An important snag of all out-patient trials of this sort is not only that the patient may not take the drugs as prescribed, but that he may also take drugs not prescribed, in which one has to include alcohol.

Promotional trials

What the pharmaceutical industry calls promotional trials must be mentioned, if only to dispel the notion that there is something sinister

DRUG EXPERIENCE REPORT

SECTION I: BASIC REACTION DATA

DATE SENT TO AUTHORITIES

day   month   year

1. ☐ INITIAL REPORT
   ☐ FOLLOW UP REPORT

2. PATIENT INITIALS AND IDENTIFICATION NUMBER

3. (leave blank)

4. SEX ☐ M ☐ F

5. HEIGHT   cm

WEIGHT   kg

6. DATE OF BIRTH
   day   month   year

7. ETHNIC GROUP:

8. DATE OF REACTION ONSET
   day   month   year

9. SOURCE OF REPORT (Mfr., Hospital, etc) (Name of reporting Physician is optional)

10. ADDRESS OF SOURCE (Give Street, City and Country)

11. DESCRIBE COMPLICATION(S) POSSIBLY ☐   PROBABLY ☐   DUE TO THE INVESTIGATIONAL DRUG(S):

12. OUTCOME OF REACTION OR COMPLICATION TO DATE
    ☐ ALIVE WITH SEQUELAE
    ☐ RECOVERED ON:
    ☐ DIED
    ☐ TREATMENT WITHDRAWN ON:
    ☐ TREATMENT CONTINUED

13. LIST ALL THERAPY IN ORDER OF SUSPICION (including self-medicated drugs)

NAME or PREP. No. of DRUG	BATCH No.	DOSAGE FORM (tab, cap, etc.)	TOTAL DAILY DOSE	ROUTE (po, im, iv, etc.)	DURATION OF THERAPY	DATES OF ADMINISTRATION	14. DISORDER OR REASON FOR USE OF DRUG

SECTION II: IMPORTANT MODIFYING DATA

15. SUBSTANTIATING LABORATORY STUDIES (Clinical Laboratory, Autopsy, X-Ray, etc.)

CLINICAL LAB: DONE ☐ NOT DONE ☐ ATTACHED ☐
BIOPSY / AUTOPSY: DONE ☐ NOT DONE ☐ ATTACHED ☐

16. LIST POTENTIALLY NOXIOUS OR ENVIRONMENTAL FACTORS (Include household products, industrial and agricultural chemicals)

17. EXISTING OR PRIOR DISORDERS AND PAST DRUG REACTION OR ALLERGIC HISTORY

PREVIOUS EXPOSURE TO SUSPECTED DRUG OR RELATED COMPOUND
☐ YES ☐ NO

18.   (a) IF FEMALE   (b) IF PREGNANT

GRAVIDITY   PARITY   WEEKS OF GESTATION

19. (leave blank)

FOR INTERNAL USE ONLY

20. REACTION FACTORS (Check all applicable boxes)
☐ DECOMPOSITION OF DRUG   ☐ INTERACTION OF TWO OR MORE DRUGS   ☐ DRUG NOT USED ACCORDING TO LABELLING   ☐ DRUG OUTDATED
☐ DRUG MISUSED BY PATIENT   ☐ OVERDOSAGE   ☐ DRUG MISLABELLED   ☐ CONTAMINATION OF DRUG   ☐ OTHER DRUG MISUSE (Specify)

72. 13. 303   Use additional sheet if necessary

FIG. 13

about them. What is usually meant, and what I mean, by a promotional trial, is the scientific investigation of the drug in the context of where it is going to be used and in the main condition it is going to be used to treat. So often the only trials of a drug at the time of marketing which get into print are really pharmacological trials and not therapeutic trials at all. For instance when investigating a drug for angina pectoris it may be essential to do haemodynamic studies or other complex investigations which are reported in a specialist journal, but what the practitioner wants to know in the end is 'how does the drug work in the context that I am likely to use it, and how can I read something about trials of the drug which I can understand?' Promotional trials and general practitioner trials are, therefore, very often synonymous.

REFERENCES

AMERICAN RHEUMATISM ASSOCIATION (1959). *Ann. rheum. Dis.* **18**, 49.

BOARDMAN, P. L. & HART, F. D. (1967). Clinical measurement of the anti-inflammatory effects of salicylates in rheumatoid arthritis. *Br. med. J.* **4**, 264.

CLARK, C. J. & DOWNIE, C. C. (1966). A method for the rapid determination of the number of patients to include in a controlled clinical trial. *Lancet*, **2**, 1357.

EMPIRE RHEUMATISM COUNCIL (1960). Initial report. *Ann. rheum. Dis.* **19**, 95.

EMPIRE RHEUMATISM COUNCIL (1961). Final report. *Ann. rheum. Dis.* **20**, 315.

HILL, A. BRADFORD (1967). *Principles of Medical Statistics.* London: Lancet.

JOYCE, C. R. B. (1968). *Psychopharmacology: Dimensions and Perspectives.* London: Tavistock.

MAXWELL, C. (1968a). The choice of design for clinical trials. *Clin. Trial J.* **5**, 1139.

MAXWELL, C. (1968b). The significance of significance. *Clin Trials,* **5**, 1015.

MEDICAL RESEARCH COUNCIL (1948). Streptomycin treatment of pulmonary tuberculosis. *Br. med. J.* **2**, 769.

MEDICAL RESEARCH COUNCIL (1950). Treatment of pulmonary tuberculosis with streptomycin and para-amino-salicylic acid. *Br. med. J.* **2**, 1073.

RITCHIE, D. M., BOYLE, J. A., MCINNES, J. M., JASANI, M. K., DALAKOS, T. G., GRIEVESON, P. & BUCHANAN, W. W. (1968). Clinical studies with an Articular Index for the assessment of joint tenderness in patients with rheumatoid arthritis. *Q. Jl Med.* **37**, 393.

ROYAL SOCIETY OF MEDICINE (1966). Measurement in therapeutic assessment. A symposium. *Proc. R. Soc. Med.* **59**, Suppl.

SWAN, H. T. & JOWETT, G. H. (1959). Treatment of iron deficiency with ferrous fumarate. Assessment by a statistically accurate method. *Br. med. J.* **2**, 782.

STATISTICAL CONSIDERATIONS IN THE DESIGN OF CLINICAL TRIALS

Cyril Maxwell

I do not mind lying, but I hate inaccuracy.
Samuel Butler, 1835-1905.

The wise, young, but perhaps inexperienced doctor usually knows of three stages to a clinical trial. He starts with the stage of design; at the end of this he embarks on the stage of execution, and at the end of this he collects his results and goes along to see a grey-haired statistician for the start of stage three—the stage of analysis.

The statistician has earned his grey hairs by being plagued by wise, young, inexperienced doctors who consult him at the end of their trial instead of at the beginning. So the statistician seizes this opportunity to teach the wise, young, inexperienced doctor his first lesson in statistics. He advises him how he should assemble his results and then tells him what he can do with them!

So the next time the wise, young, though now not quite so inexperienced doctor embarks on a clinical trial he appreciates that just as the stage of execution is considered in the design stage, so also is the stage of analysis. He therefore arranges a meeting with the statistician, this time before the trial begins.

There is, of course, only one question with which the statistician can possibly help him: ' How many patients do we need for our trial?' At this, the statistician lowers his grey-haired head five degrees and, looking over the tops of his crescent-shaped metal-rimmed spectacles, retorts: ' How good is your drug?' The excellence or otherwise of the meal which you have just finished will assist you in selecting an adjective sufficiently suitable to emphasise the wicked thought fighting its way through the alcoholic haze! ' If we knew how good the drug was, we wouldn't need to do the . . . . trial!'

It is at this stage that the wise young doctor comes to one of two conclusions. Either, one, he decides that he really must do something about finding out what statistics is all about or, two, he concludes that all statisticians are insufferable.

This paper will discuss what they might have been talking about before the trial started, had the wise young doctor only known better. There are ten headings for discussion; relevant factors, dosage, assessments, controls, significance levels, number of patients, timing of analysis, drop-outs and defaulters, documentation and trial design.

RELEVANT FACTORS

Relevant factors are those aspects of the patient, his disease and its prognosis which might affect the outcome to treatment. Some of the factors relevant to the patient include age, sex, whether he is an in-patient, an out-patient or in general practice, the personal history and many others

Of the illness, perhaps the most important are the definition of the diagnosis and the level of severity which will include it or exclude it from the trial.

Factors relevant to the prognosis include such aspects as the response to previous illnesses, the family history, the response to previous treatments and so on.

Relevant factors are those items, therefore, which describe the population in which the trial will be conducted and there are several reasons for discussing them.

Effect on distribution

The distribution in the trial may be affected by the way the population is defined. An example will illustrate this. Suppose there is a trial in hypertension. One of the things that must be agreed is the *definition* of hypertension. It would be quite reasonable to define hypertension as a patient suffering from any one (or more) of a given list of symptoms and signs in conjunction with a high systolic blood pressure. But how high?

Well, blood pressure is normally distributed. That is, if one plots actual blood pressure readings against the number of people having them (Fig. 1), the curve produced is both symmetrical and bell-shaped; it is what is called a normal distribution. There is a mean of 126 mm Hg with a standard deviation of 13.

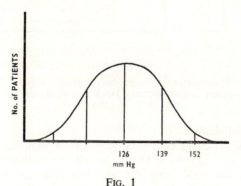

FIG. 1

Systolic blood pressure is normally distributed about a mean of 126 mm Hg. With a standard deviation of 13, only $2\frac{1}{2}$ per cent of readings lie beyond 152 mm Hg.

Now it is a property of the normal curve that only $2\frac{1}{2}$ per cent of results lie beyond the point two standard deviations above the mean (in this case, beyond 152 mm Hg), and it would be perfectly reasonable to define 'high' as being a blood pressure in excess of two standard deviations. By definition then, the distribution of the trial is no longer normal, as in Figure 1, but shaped as in Figure 2.

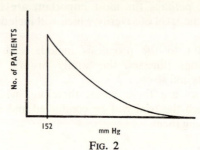

FIG. 2

If systolic pressures of less than 152 are excluded from the trial, the distribution is no longer normal.

How the statistician deals with this distribution is entirely his affair, but he has a right to know how it came about, especially when he gets the result, not as in Figure 2, but as in Figure 3.

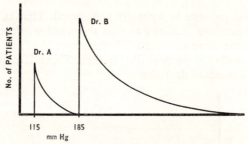

FIG. 3

The results are dichotomous because the population is dichotomous. Dr A is a paediatrician and Dr B is a geriatrician.

Modality of distribution

The unimodal curve of Figure 2 is now a bimodal curve, which happened because no-one bothered to tell the statistician that there were two doctors conducting the trial and that one of them was a paediatrician and the other was a geriatrician. The blood pressure means are, of course, quite different for the two differently aged populations. The older one is, the higher the blood pressure tends to be. Age is a relevant factor.

Randomisation

A third reason for discussing relevant factors is the randomisation. The randomisation procedure is that process by which it is determined in advance, and by random, which treatment will be given to what patient.

Single randomisation. The dispensing list (in the centre of Figure 4) pre-determines that the first patient that comes along will receive treatment A, the second B, the third B, the fourth A and so on.

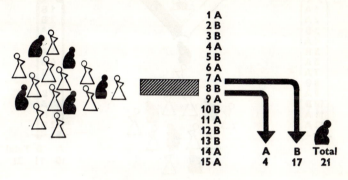

FIG. 4

The distribution of therapies amongst sub-groups is left to chance with a single (simple) randomisation.

Now it just so happens that amongst the patients coming up to the dispensing list there are some dark figures; they are dark figures because they are depressed, and these depressed patients appear in a random order. Whilst the randomisation list has been perfectly satisfactory in distributing the two treatments equally throughout the grand mass of the patients, when one comes to look specifically at the depressed patients one now finds, with dismay, that although there were 21 such patients, they did not divide equally between the two drugs; 4 had A, and 17 had B. This makes a statistical analysis very hard.

It is also a pity, for if it were known in advance that this type of analysis would be required, one could have ensured that however many there were of this particular type, half would receive one drug and half the other. Instead of using a single randomisation one would have used a stratified randomisation.

Stratified randomisation. In Figure 5, there is not one randomisation list but two. First the doctor sorts the patients into 'depressed' and 'non-depressed'. The non-depressed patients go to the left where they have a dispensing list of their own, and the depressed patients go to the right where they have their own dispensing list. At the end of the trial there are still the same 21 depressed patients, but this time they are evenly divided between the two drugs.

Note especially, that in stratifying the randomisation, one did not set out to *collect* 21 depressed patients; the purpose of the stratification was to ensure that however many there happened to be of this particular type, the treatments would be equally, though randomly, divided amongst them.

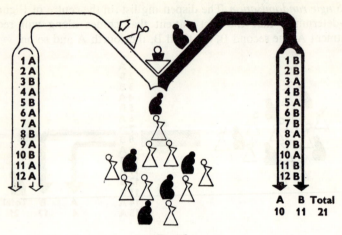

FIG. 5

A stratified randomisation ensures that the therapies are equally (though randomly) divided within each sub-group of the population.

Balanced (factorial) randomisation. There are certain types of trial in which one does set out to collect a specified number of particular types of patient. In Figure 6 it is intended to collect, with the aid of a

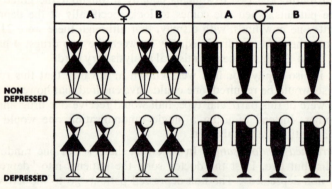

FIG. 6

The balanced (factorial) randomisation ensures that specific numbers of patients of each type are collected and that the therapies are equally spread within each 'cell'.

balanced or factorial randomisation, specific numbers of particular types of patients. In this example, it is intended to collect four female non-depressed patients, four female depressed, four male non-depressed and four male depressed patients. Furthermore, one ensures that out of each set of four, two have one treatment (randomly allocated) and two the other.

DOSAGE

Dosage may be fixed or variable. Whichever it is, it may or may not be given in conjunction with additional treatment. When additional treatment is given or when the dosage is variable, two things need discussing; the criteria for changes of dosage and the interpretation of the effect.

Criteria

Apart from the actual dose levels selected, one must define accurately the criteria for *changes* of dosage. If, say, a sore big toe is being treated (Fig. 7), one must define precisely how much worse it has to become before the dose may be increased; what is required for the dose to be maintained; how much better it has to become for the dose to be decreased; and when one must stop.

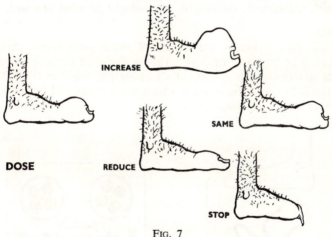

Fig. 7
Criteria must be defined accurately.

Interpretation of the effect

The way the results will be interpreted also needs discussing in relation to both the dose and the additional treatment. The big toe may have been treated with one tablet three times a day; not having got better the dose was doubled and capsules given as well (Fig. 8); now, when the toe is better one must try to decide whether this is because of the increased dose or because of the additional treatment. It is by discussing this sort of problem before the trial starts, that one avoids it.

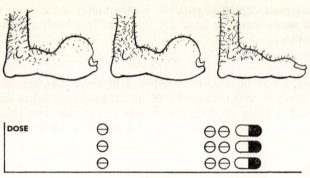

FIG. 8

What produced the cure, an increased dose or additional therapy?

ASSESSMENTS

Whose

One must make clear from whom assessments will be taken; from the patient, from the doctor, or from some auxiliary such as a biochemist, pathologist, radiologist, psychologist or what one will.

Nature

One should discuss the nature of these assessments. Are they subjective or objective or both? This is discussed because the assessments ultimately will go into the melting pot together (Fig. 9), and one needs to decide beforehand which assessments will be given most credence in cases of disagreement.

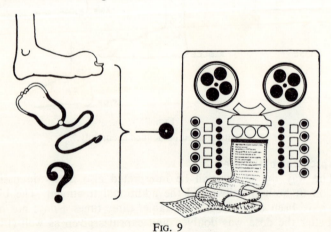

FIG. 9

The melting pot is very sophisticated nowadays.

Usually one finds that whilst the patient's assessment is predominantly subjective, the doctor's assessment is not objective enough for there is always some degree of subjectivity about the most 'objective' of assessments.

And do not dismiss too lightly the importance of this. One must counterbalance the Hamiltonian view: 'never believe a word the patient tells you', with the Maxwellian view: 'doctors are in business to relieve suffering and the best judge of suffering is the sufferer'! Clearly, both of these are extremes and the correct attitude lies somewhere between the two.

Type of measurement

The type of measurement must be discussed. Are the assessments *interval* variety, *nominal* variety or *ordinal*?

There are three types of measurement (Fig. 10). There is interval measurement such as with a ruler where the difference between two adjacent marks on the measure are the same as the difference between any other two adjacent marks. There is nominal measurement in which one classifies or categorises what one is measuring into broad arbitrary groups such as 'large', 'medium' and 'small'. And there is ordinal measurement in which they are placed in an ascending or descending order; largest, second largest, third, fourth and so on.

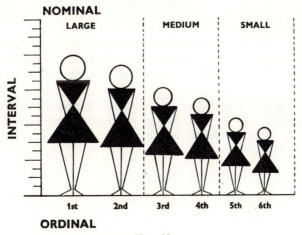

FIG. 10

Three types of measurement.

Often the type of measurement determines the most suitable type of statistical test; the best known being the 't' test for interval measurement, the χ^2 test for nominal measurement, and a variety of tests including the Rank-Sign test, the Mann-Whitney 'U' test, the Wilcoxon matched-pairs, and many others for ordinal measurement.

Transformations

One should discuss whether transformations are necessary. Statisticians like working with normal type curves and they are prepared to go to apparently extraordinary lengths to obtain them. They can often convert a ' skewed' curve (obtained perhaps by measuring with an ordinary ruler) into a normal curve by transforming the units into, say, log units (Fig. 11).

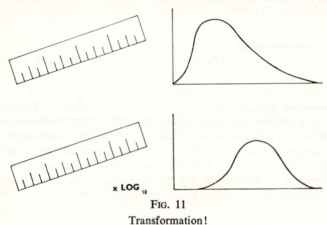

× LOG₁₀

Fig. 11
Transformation!

Timing

Finally, one must consider the timing of the assessments. These must be done when they will best show the differences that are being sought. Are the assessments to be made daily, or weekly, or monthly, or when?

Often, a before-and-after assessment is all that is required. If one is comparing *rates* of response, more frequent assessments will be necessary, whilst if one is recording attacks or incidents, continual recording will be necessary.

CONTROLS

The control may be either no-treatment, a placebo (which is *not* the same) or an active treatment. Whichever it is, the control needs to have certain properties, particularly validity and suitability.

Validity

The control needs to have validity in relation to the question that the trial is set up to answer. It must be a fair comparison. For example, if the new treatment is an anti-depressant and an active control is wanted it would be wrong to select an antibiotic. An antibiotic would not be a valid control. Put another way, if one is comparing Stork with butter, one must have the right Stork! (Fig. 12).

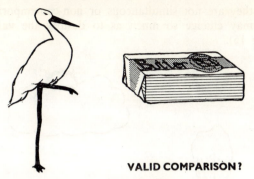

VALID COMPARISON?

FIG. 12

Suitability

Just as it needs to be a fair or valid comparison, so also does it need to be a competent one. For example, if one is designing a control to compare a new treatment's speed of action, a no-treatment control would be ridiculous (Fig. 13).

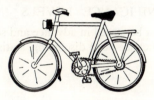

WHICH IS FASTER?

FIG. 13

Contemporaneousness

The time relationship between the control and the trial therapy may be of importance. If the control and the trial therapy are given simultaneously, external conditions can be presumed to be constant (Fig. 14);

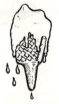

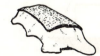

FIG. 14

Simultaneous control . . .

whereas if they are not simultaneous or non-contemporary, external conditions may change so much as to destroy the validity of the control (Fig. 15).

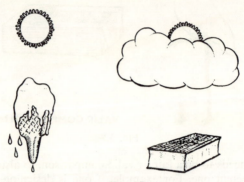

FIG. 15
... or control at a different time?

SIGNIFICANCE LEVELS

Significance levels must be stated in advance and set before the trial starts. Two types of significance need discussing, statistical significance and clinical significance.

Statistical significance

One should discuss in advance of the trial, alpha, two-alpha, beta and 1−beta.

Alpha is the probability of a Type 1 statistical error. It is the probability of finding a difference when no such difference actually exists. It is the probability of a false positive result (Fig 16).

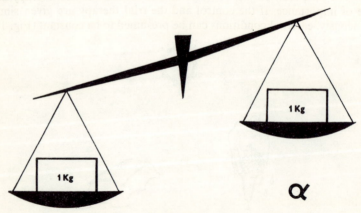

FIG. 16
Alpha is the probability of a Type I error.

Because exactly the same error can occur in the opposite direction (Fig. 17), it is necessary to discuss alpha times two or two-alpha.

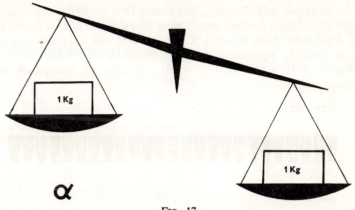

FIG. 17
The Type I error can go two ways.

A converse type of error is the Type 2 statistical error; the probability of which is beta. Beta is the probability of finding no difference where there really is one. It is the probability of a false negative result (Fig. 18). It is thus a measure of the sensitivity of the statistical test, which is discussed in typically inverse manner by statisticians as 1 − beta, which is known as the ' power of the test '.

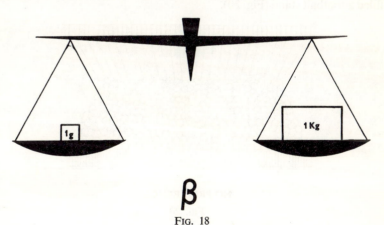

FIG. 18
Beta is the probability of a Type II error.

Clinical significance

Clinical significance is the worthwhileness of the treatment in purely medical terms, and it is entirely arbitrary. It is nothing to do with probablity or chance or mathematics. One should discuss under this heading the size of the difference between the therapies and the total sample size, usually designated as ' N '.

An example will illustrate this point. In a northern city recently people attending a football match were asked which of two teams was best. Very many more thought ' City ' was best and this result (Fig. 19) was statistically significant at the 0·001 level. There was only one chance in a thousand of this result occurring by chance. A very impressive result!

CITY BEST

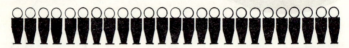

UNITED BEST

p<·001

FIG. 19

What tended to spoil it was the number of people who could not tell a difference between the two. They were so numerous that they filled a football stand (Fig. 20).

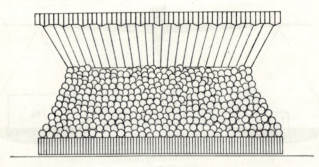

NO PREFERENCE

FIG. 20

NUMBERS OF PATIENTS

One must discuss the numbers of patients required to yield a meaningful result. It will be recognised that the introduction to this paper was facetious. In actual fact, one often does have an idea of how potent a therapy is, and when this is so there are graphs (Fig. 21) published by Clark and Downie (1966) which help, provided also one has an idea of how the control group might respond.

NUMBER OF PATIENTS REQUIRED FOR CLINICAL TRIALS

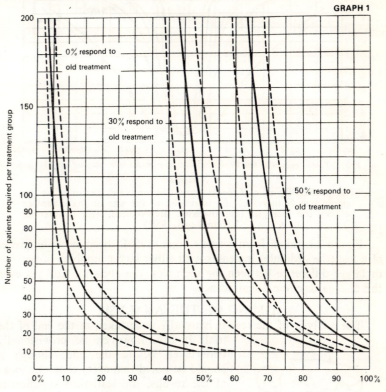

FIG. 21

Number of patients required for a clinical trial when the expected response to established treatment is 0, 30 or 50 per cent. (Reproduced, with permission, from Clark and Downie, 1966.)

There are also tables published elsewhere by the author (1968) which look like a crib but are not; these have also been calculated on an electronic computer but by a different technique and these figures are more cautious.

On the other hand, one may have no clue about potency in that particular population, and then one must guess. When making a guess one should consider the self-imposed level of clinical significance for in the long run, it is this that really matters.

Regardless of whether or not one has a reliable guide to the number of patients. one needs to discuss the numbers of patients (N), in relation to alpha, beta, and the size of the difference between the therapies, for these are all inter-related with each other.

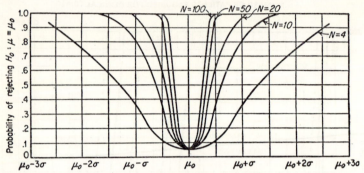

FIG. 1. Power curves of the two-tailed test at α = .05 with varying sample sizes.

FIG. 22

The probability of a Type II error (the ordinate) decreases as the sample size N increases and is related to the size of the difference between the therapies (the abscissa). (Reproduced, with permission, from Siegel, 1956.)

Figure 22, taken from Siegel's book (1956), shows how the power of a test (the ordinate) increases with either larger numbers of patients or larger difference between the therapies (the abcissa). And yet even this disregards *clinical* significance.

TIMING OF THE ANALYSIS

The analysis of the results is usually undertaken at the end of the trial. It can, however, be provisionally undertaken before the end, though it should be noted that every time one looks at the results, the statistical significance level being taken as meaningful, needs to be made more strict.

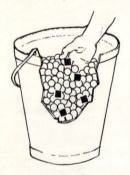

FIG. 23

There are five false positive results in every hundred. The more often one looks, the greater the chance of picking one out.

The reason for this is because by definition, at the 0·05 level of significance, there are five false-positive results in every hundred. There are five chances in a hundred of finding a so-called 'difference' when no such difference really exists, and the more often one looks at the results (Fig. 23) the greater is the chance of picking one of these out by accident.

There is a special technique by which the results can be analysed as one goes along. This is the sequential trial. The results are charted as they become available on a special chart, one example of which is shown in Figure 24. One starts on the black square and every time a preference is obtained, a cross is made in the square immediately above or to the right of the last one depending on the direction of the preference. As soon as one of the boundaries is crossed, the trial stops.

SEQUENTIAL CHART

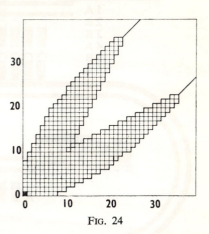

FIG. 24

DROP-OUTS AND DEFAULTERS

Drop-outs and defaulters are those patients who enter the trial but, for any of a wide variety of reasons, never finish it.

One should try to anticipate their effect on the randomisation. With single and stratified randomisations, it is not usually necessary to adjust the randomisation procedure, but with balanced (factorial) randomisations it is essential to replace patients who default (Fig. 25) or one will end up with incomplete cells.

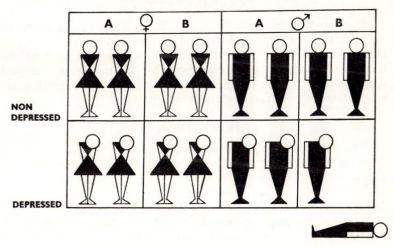

FIG. 25

In balanced (factorial) designs drop-outs must be replaced.

If they are numerous, one must consider whether it may be worthwhile interpreting the drop-outs in their own right. The purpose of the randomisation is to put equal numbers of passengers on to two trains

(Fig. 26). If one of the trains arrives almost empty, this in itself may be meaningful.

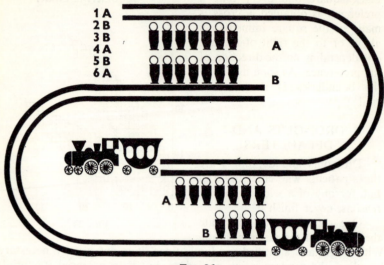

FIG. 26

This needs explaining. Why did one train lose so many passengers?

DOCUMENTATION

One should discuss with the statistician, and in very full detail, all the documents for the trial: dispensing lists, prescription forms, progress chasers and especially assessment sheets, with regard to both the number of documents and their layout; for whilst they are designed specifically for the convenience of the investigator, it is the statistician who is required to extract the data from them (Fig. 27).

TRIAL DESIGN

The choice of design for our scientific experiment can be made from the following: matched pairs, comparative groups, cross-over or mixed.

Matched pairs

Identical patients are brought together in pairs, one patient is exposed to one treatment and the other patient exposed to the other treatment. This is shown diagrammatically in Figure 28 as patients entering two arks. The difference between these two arks (representing treatments) and Noah's is that, whilst the animals go in two-by-two, these pairs are absolutely identical even for sex.

The disadvantages of this type of trial are two-fold. The matching must be perfect and one does not always know which factors are

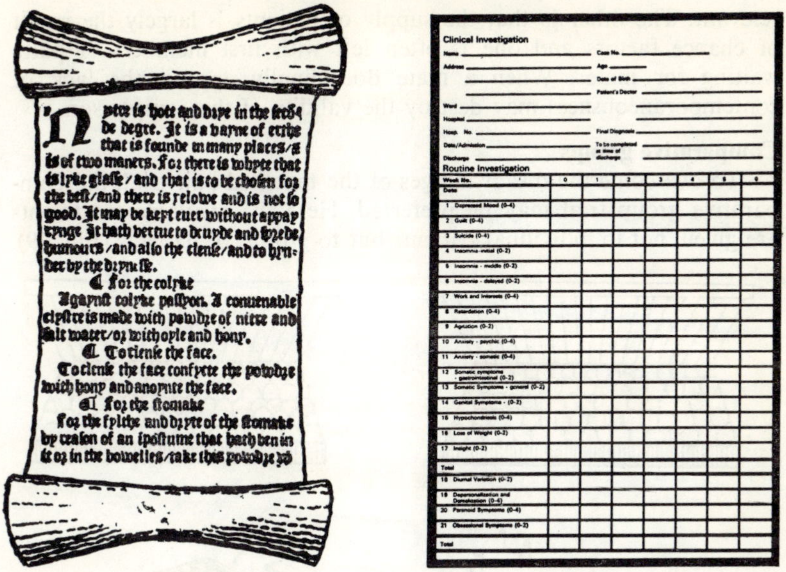

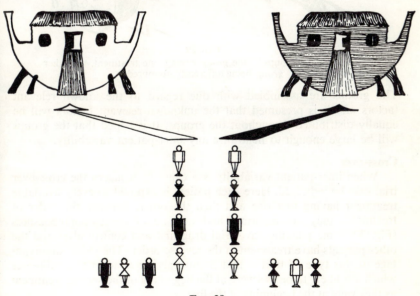

FIG. 27
Both will do the job. One will do it easier.

FIG. 28
'Matched pairs.'. The animals go in two-by-two and are absolutely identical,
even for sex. One member of the pair goes into one treatment (ark) and the
other takes the alternative. Note that six patients (at the bottom) are not yet
'matched', is there a problem here?

relevant. The other is that the supply of patients is largely the result of chance factors and one is often left with first members of pairs waiting for mates. When a mate does finally appear, the lack of contemporaneousness may destroy the validity of the comparison.

Comparative groups

To overcome the disadvantages of the matched pair trial, the comparative group trial may be preferred. Here the available treatments are given, not to individual patients but to *groups* of patients (Fig. 29).

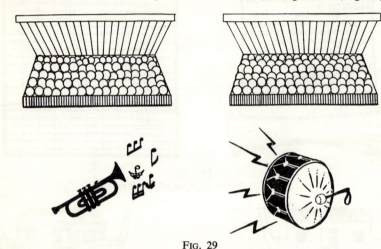

FIG. 29

'Comparative groups'. One *group* having one treatment, the other *group* being differently honoured.

The groups are assembled with due regard to the known relevant factors and it is presumed that the unknown relevant factors will be equally distributed throughout the groups. It is hoped that the groups will be large enough to neutralise any inter-patient variability.

Cross-over

When inter-patient variability is a cause for concern the cross-over trial may be indicated. Here each patient is exposed to every available treatment having first one and then the other. Because the order of treatments may be important and because of contemporaneousness (Fig. 30) some patients have trial drug first and control after and the other patients have treatment in the reverse order. The major disadvantage of this type of trial is that it can only be done in those diseases which are likely to be as severe at the beginning of the second treatment as they were at the beginning of the first.

Mixed designs

Each type of design has its faults but these can often be minimised by mixing the trial designs. One could mix a matched pair design with a cross-over or one could do a cross-over in comparative groups and so on. Whichever design is selected, however, the statistician must be fully informed so that errors in statistical thinking can be identified before it is too late.

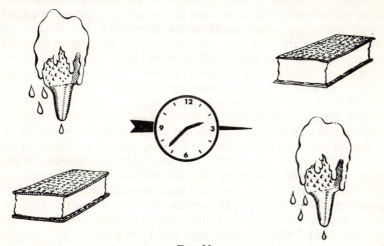

FIG. 30
' Cross-over '. No matter which comes first, the cone still melts faster.

CONCLUSION

The essence of collaboration with a statistician lies in the conference before the trial starts. This is the time when errors can be identified and something constructive done about them. This is the time to invite criticism for later may be too late. Always remember that the final invitation to criticism is the publication of the results and the swine that writes that searching letter to the editor may be me!

ACKNOWLEDGEMENTS

I am grateful to Dr C. C. Downie and the *Lancet* for permission to publish Figure 21, and to the McGraw-Hill Book Company Inc., for permission to publish Figure 22.

I am extremely grateful to Dr R Ollerenshaw and the Department of Medical Illustration of the University of Manchester for the preparation of the slides and figures, and to Dr Ollerenshaw for much helpful advice in the construction of this lecture.

REFERENCES

CLARK, C. J. & DOWNIE, C. C. (1966). A method for the rapid determination of the number of patients to include in a controlled clinical trial. *Lancet* **2,** 1357.
MAXWELL, C. (1968). The significance of significance. *Clin. Trial* 5, 1015.
SIEGEL, S. (1956). *Non-parametric Statistics for the Behavioural Sciences.* London: McGraw Hill.

FURTHER READING

I have been asked to produce a list of references for further reading and so as not to disappoint the hard-working editors, a list is dutifully appended at the end of this section. This list will be invaluable to those with abundant funds who are endeavouring to ensure that their library shelves are complete. If on the other hand, dear reader, you are groping in the dark and wondering where to go from here, let me see if I can help you. I will presume that you are completely ignorant of statistics and relatively unaware of clinical trial design (that is, of course, with the exception of the pearls of wisdom you have picked up on your journey to this page!).

But first, a general word of advice. Like the foreigner learning English, you will discover that clinical trials are extremely easy to do if you do not mind doing them badly; they are rather difficult to do well. Statistics do not even offer the consolation of simplicity at any price. If you wish to develop only an *understanding* of the relevant statistical procedures, you will still need to work fairly hard and to persevere even when all looks hopeless. But do not despair, it can be done, and in not too long a time. For you, dear reader, are less ignorant than I was five years ago, and I am going to give you the benefit of my experience to stop you deviating down paths of utter irrelevance and even greater bewilderment. Follow my advice and you will develop an understanding of the principles in a matter of a few weeks.

Just as with any other subject, it is impossible to prepare one publication that is at the same time simple to comprehend, easy to read, assuming no great knowledge of the reader, and yet fully comprehensive. Thus I am unable to recommend any *one* book to you and say that it contains just what you want. Some come rather near to this ideal but none is without its disadvantages.

How about a very short introduction to start with? Have a look at *The Clinical Trial's Protocol* (Maxwell, 1969) and read the chapter entitled 'Very elementary statistics'. Another one on the 'Choice of design' might be helpful. You might find the other chapters useful, and they will not take you long to read.

When you have done this, I will ask you to invest in three books by Smart (1963), Hamilton (1961) and Hill (1966), and these will be the most useful books you will have bought on the subject. I think you will find yourself buying others that I mention, but I want you to order these three first, for at any level of learning they are invaluable.

Now, dear reader, I am going to ask you to do something unusual. Please do not open these three books. Put them on your book shelf and wait.

First, I want you to borrow Siegel (1956) and read only the first 34 pages (chapters 1 to 3 inclusive). You must not read any more, though I do not mind you turning over the pages if you like. You will probably find the format so attractive that you will want to buy it, but do not read beyond this point yet.

Now on your bookshelf are three slender volumes, two of which can be read very quickly. Why not whip through Smart (1963) very quickly; do not spend too much time with the calculations, just get an impression of the jargon and the different applications of the various tests. Do not try to read it as a textbook, it is too good for that. Try and read it in a few evenings. Do not worry at this stage if you are not retaining it. You have paid for the book and it is yours, you can always come back to it later—and you will!

Now read Hamilton (1961) in very much the same way. There is no reason to take too long on this slim volume, for these are the lectures you wished you had had when you were a student. But now you get them without the discomfort of note-taking and a hard seat, and you will come back to them time and time again.

' What,' you may ask, ' about the other one?' Can you skim through Bradford Hill (Hill, 1966)? The answer is that you can, but you will kick yourself afterwards if you do. You *can* get away with just reading the summaries at the end of each chapter. But you will be missing the opportunity of a lifetime if you do, because you are now at a stage when you will be able to learn for all time the basic fundamental principles on which good clinical trials are based. Start at the very beginning and do not turn a page until you have understood exactly what you have read. You should have no difficulty, for it is written with a logic beyond reproach. There are some chapters (XVII-XIX) which can be safely omitted but do not avoid any of the rest.

By now you will have gone through Smart, Hamilton and Bradford Hill and you will probably feel that although Bradford Hill has dealt superbly with parametric statistics, it has not really gone into those non-parametric tests that Smart described briefly. Well, you will find those in Siegel (1956). I do not recommend that you *read* Siegel (apart from the early chapters which I mentioned above), but it is a most perfect reference book for non-parametric statistics and one which can be browsed through happily.

Up till now you have been reading how to develop an understanding of the statistical procedures involved in clinical trials. If you want to become a statistician, you will need more sophisticated books (some of which are listed at the end), but at this stage you will probably be wanting to get back to clinical trials.

To recommend general reading on clinical trials is not easy (indeed, that is the main justification for *this* book). The best and most appropriate reading is dependent on what you are looking for and I would suggest that you first decide what it is that you are looking for and then try the indexes or lists of contents (or in the case of papers, the summaries) or some of those in the following list. But first a word of advice.

Approaching a new subject is always difficult but you, dear reader, have friends and allies. You will find as I have done that everyone involved with them is anxious that clinical trials should become better and better. Because of this, and because they are good chaps as well, they will be only too happy to give you the benefit of their experience. Do not hesitate to pick their brains and ask them for help, for in so doing both will benefit.

REFERENCES

Essential reading

HAMILTON, M. (1961). *Lectures on the Methodology of Clinical Research.* Edinburgh: Livingstone.

HILL, A. BRADFORD (1966). *Principles of Medical Statistics,* 8th ed. London: Lancet.

MAXWELL, C. (1969). *The Clinical Trials Protocol: A Primer For Clinical Trials.* London: Clinical Trials Journal.

SIEGEL, S. (1956). *Non-parametric Statistics for the Behavioural Sciences.* London: McGraw-Hill.

SMART, J. V. (1963). *Elements of Medical Statistics.* London: Staples Press.

Statistics

ARMITAGE, P. (1960). *Sequential Medical Trials.* Oxford: Blackwell.

BENJAMIN, B. (1959). *Elements of Vital Statistics.* London: Allen and Unwin.

DAVIES, O. L. (1957). *Statistical Methods in Research and Production.* Edinburgh: Oliver and Boyd.

DAVIES, O. L. (1954). *The Design and Analysis of Industrial Experiments.* I.C.I. Monograph. Edinburgh: Oliver and Boyd.

FISHER, R. A. (1954). *Statistical Methods for Research Workers,* 12th ed. Edinburgh: Oliver and Boyd.

FISHER, R. A. (1951). *The Design of Experiments,* 6th ed. Edinburgh: Oliver and Boyd.

FISHER, R. A. & YATES, F. (1963). *Statistical Tables for Biological, Agricultural and Medical Research.* Edinburgh: Oliver and Boyd.

HERDAN, G. (1955). *Statistics of Therapeutic Trials.* Amsterdam: Elsevier.

HILL, A. BRADFORD (1962). *Statistical Methods in Clinical and Preventive Medicine.* Edinburgh: Livingstone.

HUFF, DARREL (1954). *How to Lie with Statistics.* London: Gollancz.

MAINLAND, D. (1963). *Elementary Medical Statistics.* Philadelphia: Saunders.

MAXWELL, A. E. (1961). *Analysing Qualitative Data.* London: Methuen.

MORONEY, M. J. (1963). *Facts From Figures.* London: Penguin.

QUENOUILLE, M. H. (1959). *Rapid Statistical Calculations.* London: Griffin.

SNEDECOR, G. W. (1962). *Statistical Methods Applied to Experiments in Agriculture and Biology.* Iowa: The Iowa State University Press.

STIBITZ, G. R. (1966). *Mathematics in Medicine and the Life Sciences.* Chicago: Year Book Medical Publishers.

Clinical trials

HILL, A. BRADFORD (1960). *Controlled Clinical Trials.* Oxford: Blackwell.

LAURENCE, D. R. & BACHARACH, A. L. (1964). *Evaluation of Drug Activities—Pharmacometrics,* Vols 1 and 2. New York: Academic Press.

LONG, E. A. (1967). *Clinical Trials—a Report to the Association of the British Pharmaceutical Industry.* London: The Association of the British Pharmaceutical Industry.

MAINLAND, D. (1960). *The clinical trial—some difficulties and suggestions.* *J. Chron. Dis.* **11**, 484.

MAINLAND, D. (1960). The use and misuse of statistics in medical publications. *Clin. Pharmac. Ther.* **1**, 411.

MODELL, W. (1960). Anyone for a symposium? *Clin. Pharmac. Ther.* **1**, 689.

NODINE, J. H. & SIEGLER, P. E. (1964 & 1967). *Animal and Clinical Pharmacologic Techniques in Drug Evaluation* Vols 1 and 2. Chicago: Year Book Medical Publishers.

SAINSBURY, P. & KREITMAN, N. S. (1963). *Methods of Psychiatric Research.* London: Oxford University Press.

WAIFE, S. O. & SHAPIRO, A. P. (1959). *The Clinical Evaluation of New Drugs.* New York: Hoeber-Harper.

WITTS, L. J. (1959). *Medical Surveys and Clinical Trials.* London: Oxford University Press.

WORLD HEALTH ORGANISATION (1968). Principles for the clinical evaluation of drugs. *Wld Hlth Org. Tech. Rep. Ser.* No. 403.

ZAIMIS, E. & ELIS, J. (1965). *Evaluation of New Drugs in Man.* Oxford: Pergamon Press.

CLINICAL TRIALS—
PRACTICAL AND COMMERCIAL CONSIDERATIONS

T. B. BINNS

This paper is concerned with various aspects of trials that are not dealt with elsewhere in this book. They will be discussed under the following headings: (1) background influences, (2) effect of drug control authorities, (3) considerations for prospective trialists, such as assessment of laboratory data and use of resources and (4) payment for trials.

Background influences

Only recently was it reported that expenditure on the National Health Service has at last risen above 5 per cent of the national income (*Medical Tribune,* 6 February, 1969). It always seems astonishing that as a nation we allow the politicians to spend, relatively speaking, so little on health and in particular on therapeutics, since I cling to the belief that most people go to their doctors to be made better. Many medical schools still give comparatively low priority to both teaching and research in therapeutics and though most doctors would agree that modern prescribing is greatly influenced by clinical trials, the vast majority of them are quite prepared to leave these to others.

Hence, for the profession, clinical trials remain of peripheral and secondary importance, even in the area of research. For industry, on the other hand, it has rapidly become obvious that clinical trials stand right in the path of drug development. They are of crucial importance because they verify the validity or otherwise of all the previous research; and they enable Management to make important decisions on whether and how to market a drug. A complete and accurate picture is needed as expeditiously as possible.

There are alarming but apparently inexorable trends, which cause economic rather than scientific or humanitarian considerations increasingly to influence the type of compound which is looked for and which ultimately comes forward for trial. Industry realises the need to develop preparations that contribute to medical progress, but no firm can afford to allocate a high proportion of its research effort to basic work with no foreseeable therapeutic application. The prospects of success are too remote (Bloch and Paget, 1968). The search for useful new drugs is steadily becoming technically more difficult and economically more hazardous. It usually takes five to seven years and upwards of a million pounds to develop and market a new drug and it may be overtaken by a competitor before it ever shows a profit.

In these circumstances who is going to look for drugs for rare diseases? Nowadays they are almost always the result of an unexpected fluke. In future it is doubtful if even the flukes will ever be marketed, because it is no longer economic to develop them. One can visualise the time when governments will have to subsidise the industry to work in certain areas.

Even the large markets will no longer be attractive if success immediately leads to applications for compulsory licences under Section 41 of the Patents Act, which enable other firms to compete without capital expenditure or risk. This would mean the prompt demise of the industry as we know it. Certainly we must consider the cost and risk of progress; but we must also consider the much more imponderable cost and risk of no progress.

Naturally the therapeutic promise of a new drug is reflected in the reception given to it by prospective trialists, and it is not surprising that it is much easier to get trials done on the more exciting compounds. For reasons already described, the investment in any drug that reaches the stage of clinical trial is already so great that there is understandable reluctance to abandon the doubtful ones without good evidence. Few people are aware how much progress the biologists have already made, but there is undoubtedly a need for further refinement in the preclinical and early clinical testing of drugs so that the limited resources for extended trials are used to the best advantage.

Drug control authorities

Drug control authorities are also having an increasing effect on drug development and on the conduct of clinical trials. Although details may differ, the general principles now apply to an increasing number of countries and there is increasing interchange between them. The most important of these principles is that the responsibility for demonstrating and maintaining quality, safety and efficacy remains with the manufacturer, but the onus is on the doctor to prescribe wisely (Cahal, 1968).

It already seems almost incredible that as recently as 1963 there were no restrictions on the marketing of drugs in Britain. Our Drug Control Authority, known to everyone as the Dunlop Committee, came into operation in 1964 on a voluntary basis and was given legal status in 1968 under the Medicines Act. The system and the relationships it has built up have become a model and the envy of many other countries. One must hope that the Medicines Commission will have the vision and wisdom to preserve and build on these excellent foundations.

The secret of its undoubted success is its readiness to apply first-class professional judgement rather than a book of rules. The Committee exercises this judgement at two stages in the development of a drug; first at the end of the pre-clinical stage before clinical trials can begin, and second at the end of clinical trials before the drug can be put on the market.

Both these submissions are divided into two parts. Outlines of the proposed clinical studies are included in the clinical trials submission and are considered in relation to the other data available.

Permission to start trials may be applied for and granted stepwise. Unofficially there is a fair amount of international agreement on the duration of clinical testing that is justified by limited toxicity tests (Table I). For a new compound, even if it has already been tested elsewhere, permission in Britain is likely to be restricted to three centres, and other conditions such as the number of patients and the duration of treatment may also be imposed. This is vastly preferable to having to complete long-term toxicity tests before the drug can be given to man at all, for it is now widely accepted that these cannot be designed rationally until its metabolism in man can be compared with that in laboratory animals. Hence the whole procedure should be integrated as closely as possible.

TABLE I

Duration of toxicity and clinical testing

Clinical	Animals
Single dose	1 week[a] 3 weeks[b]
Up to 1 week	1 month
Over 1 week[a] Up to 1 month[b]	3 months
Over 1 month[b]	6 months

[a] European Society Study Drug Toxicity
[b] ABPI Expert Committee
[c] WHO Expert Committee—no specific recommendations

These requirements are exacting and the need to comply with them has undoubtedly imposed on the industry a greater need to systematise and document its work. This, of course, is all to the good, but excessive restrictions could completely inhibit progress. The problem is to keep the right balance. In some countries, repeated submissions are declared inadequate for reasons that look increasingly like bureaucratic procrastination. When this starts to happen, drug firms soon begin to wonder whether even a promising compound is worth the candle.

Any controls of this sort inevitably cause some delay and inflexibility. To keep these to a minimum it is highly desirable that investigators, and particularly acknowledged experts, should be allowed the maximum freedom of action on the basis of mutual understanding and trust between all three parties. Although it has no officially approved list of investigators, the Dunlop Committee makes no secret of its interest in who conducts the trials, especially in the early stages. It also requires that all the available information should be provided to investigators, and that any important adverse effects found by one will be notified to the others.

It seems fair to say that, with certain misgivings about the future, the industry has welcomed the added protection and help of the Committee. Its aims are not only to minimise risks, but to raise standards; those of public understanding as well as of scientific and clinical competence. Standards have certainly risen, though it is difficult to know how to apportion the credit.

Still harder to judge are two other possible effects of control authorities. The first is that they may tend to stereotype both preclinical and clinical testing along lines already known to be acceptable. Although improved tests are needed at every stage, the use of a new and possibly inadequately validated test could mean difficulty or delay in getting approval. Hence facilities and manpower might be absorbed by routine work while the more creative talent would be frustrated and go elsewhere.

The second is on the availability of compounds that are used in man largely for research purposes as diagnostic or pharmacological tools. Most firms have a few preparations that they keep in their lists, often at a loss, as a service to the profession. This type of service is becoming progressively harder to maintain.

Finally, though it is no part of the official drug control procedure, many organisations also require prior approval of all clinical research projects by a panel of competent, but non-involved, scientists. This is particularly important in certain types of study, such as those utilising normal volunteers, the mentally subnormal or children.

Considerations for prospective trialists

Assessment of laboratory data. It will probably be most helpful to look at some of the practical considerations from the viewpoint of the prospective clinical trialist, who is approached after the stage of clinical pharmacology has been completed.

The earlier in the drug's history, the more important it is for a clinician to be able to assess for himself the data already available. In the present context he will be fortified by knowing that the task will already have been undertaken by the Drug Control Authority and by one or more clinical pharmacologists, but that does not absolve him of responsibility. What then is the drug's present status? The firm's medical adviser who is monitoring the preparation is the person most likely to have a broad knowledge of it. He may want to bring in one or more of his laboratory colleagues to discuss special aspects, and the clinician considering a trial should not hesitate to ask for other advice if he needs it. Some of the most important points to look for are listed in Table II.

TABLE II

Data to be assessed by a prospective trialist
(for discussion see text)

Pharmacology
  Evidence of therapeutic promise
  Other effects

Toxicity
  Type, reversibility
  Histology
  Biochemistry
  Haematology

Metabolism
  Animals c.f. man

Clinical
  Pharmacology and toxicity

Experimental material
  Presentation, stability, etc.

Chemical similarity by no means implies biological similarity either in efficacy or toxicity, but is there evidence of therapeutic promise, especially biological activity that is novel in type or degree? What other pharmacological actions does the compound have? Are any important drug interactions foreseen?

The toxicity tests are usually deliberately planned to give clear-cut effects at the highest dose, and these are consequently to be expected, but what *type* of effect was seen and to what extent was it reversible? What histological and what haematological and biochemical effects were found? All these can give important clues to clinical toxicity. In considering the therapeutic ratio the extent of the risk that is acceptable depends very much on the circumstances. Incidentally the original toxicity tests on aspirin were confined to one fish and two frogs. So we have come a long way since then.

What information is available on the distribution and metabolism of the compound, e.g. from autoradiography with labelled drug possibly coupled with extraction and thin layer chromatography? Can it all be accounted for, and if not why? What evidence is there that the drug behaves similarly in man? What is its half-life in man compared with animals? What are the results of dose-finding and other preliminary clinical studies? Is there any evidence of clinical toxicity? For a fuller discussion reference should be made to Goldberg (1965), Paget (1965) and Spinks (1965).

Use of resources. It is an important function of the medical adviser to study the various attributes of an experimental compound and to devise a series of investigations that will shed light on their possible clinical application. The prospective trialist will consider any proposal, whatever its source, in relation to his own special circumstances. Broadly speaking the types of study that may be contemplated fall into one or more of the following categories:

1. Additional clinico-pharmacological work to elucidate the drug's mechanism of action, its effect and behaviour in the body;

2. Comparative studies against placebo or preferably against the best preparation(s) currently available for the purpose;

3. Uncontrolled ' clinical experience '.

Although well designed and conducted studies in the second category are generally the most valuable in providing reliable clinical information, the third is not to be despised. Provided that the information is properly sought and recorded, it can be used to build up a body of clinical experience, not only on tolerability but possibly also on optimum dosage regimes, new indications, etc. which can subsequently be subjected to formal trial. It is always wise for an investigator to handle a drug for a while to get the feel of it before embarking on a formal trial and in many cases pilot trials are essential. The combined views of several experienced clinicians often give an accurate preliminary impression of a new drug's value and limitations.

Unfortunately it remains a world-wide problem that clinical material and facilities for studying it are available in inverse proportion. Clinical trials cannot make a bad drug into a good one, but they certainly can fail to do a good one justice. The important thing is to make the best use of any given situation. This requires experience and judgement for ' if you wait until you can do a trial perfectly, you will probably never do it at all.' (Binns and Butterfield, 1964).

In the finality the questions that will have to be answered are: how can the best use be made of available resources to conduct a study that is still within practical limits? Is the study ethically justified and is the outcome likely to be worth the effort?

Details of design are dealt with elsewhere, but there are certain practical points that will bear emphasis or repetition. Perhaps the greatest temptation is to be too ambitious in the size, duration and scope of a trial. One should always be pessimistic about the number of patients likely to be available, but unless one is looking for minor differences, the numbers required to demonstrate *efficacy* are reasonably small.

On the other hand *tolerability* is another matter. We are interested firstly to detect any adverse reaction and secondly if possible to establish its incidence. To do this very much larger numbers of cases are required and the data should desirably be collected specially for the purpose. With pharmacogenetics in mind, it should include, for example, ethnic origin. The problem is particularly acute if the reaction occurs rarely but is serious. Although all adverse reactions on new products are supposed to be reported to the Dunlop Committee during their first two years, no entirely satisfactory way of collecting this numerator/denominator type of information has yet been devised. One could visualise a system of pre-and post-marketing vigilance that could be adjusted, like quality control in a factory, according to the need and gradually relaxed if accumulating experience was favourable.

Unfortunately it is the exception rather than the rule for adequate techniques of measurement to be available. In fact, one can state a maxim that trials of every new compound show up inadequacies in the trials of its predecessors. This can also be taken as a sign of progress.

Obviously the more subjective the criteria of assessment, the more rigid the controls have to be. Equally obviously objective criteria are useless if they are not relevant to the problem in hand. As Bradford Hill (1966) said in his Heberden oration: ' Given the right attitude of mind there is more than one way in which we can study therapeutic efficacy. Any belief that the controlled trial is the only way would mean, not that the pendulum had swung too far, but that it had come right off its hook.'

Since trials are immensely care and time consuming, it is necessary to consider at the outset who else is likely to be involved among both medical and ancillary staff and to be sure of their full support. It is good that laboratory staff, among others, upon whom so much depends, are increasingly being brought in as full participants.

Firms can do a great deal to improve the practicality and efficiency of trials by providing special packs, labels and codes.

Of course, sufficient material, both in quality and quantity, must be available. It is catastrophic to run out of stock. In some circumstances it may be necessary to ensure that it all comes from the same batch, and it is highly desirable that trials should be done with the final dosage form. If there are formulation and stability problems this may be difficult to arrange. It is also wise to try to ensure that the patient actually consumes the medicament according to directions. The incidence of defaulting can be so high that one sometimes wonders if everyone is either a placebo reactor or a defaulter, or even whether it is possible to be both! Ideally one should perform spot tests on the urine of patients, but unfortunately even qualitative tests are rarely possible. There is a considerable need for detectable inert tablet markers that would reflect the amount of drug in the body. Meanwhile, simple pill counting checks are usually the best we can manage.

Incidentally, experimental material is usually sent out on the tacit understanding that the investigator will keep the firm informed of his results and that he will be free to publish at his own discretion.

Payment for trials

This is a perennial problem which excites all shades of opinion because it is not easy to reconcile two obvious but conflicting precepts.

1. It is clearly wrong that payment, either direct or indirect, should influence the conduct of a trial or the conclusions drawn from it.

2. On the other hand it is unreasonable to expect doctors to give their advice and devote all the skill and time required without reward, when the firm stands to benefit whatever the outcome of a properly executed trial.

No one is likely to think it is improper for a firm to reimburse expenses directly incurred during the course of a trial. These may vary from paying patients' bus fares and loss of earnings resulting from special attendance, to stationery and overtime for a statistician, secretary or technician.

Likewise a modest fee for the completing of a record form for the firm's benefit would probably not be objectionable, since this would not represent payment for the trial itself, but only for the chore of the clerical work. Beyond this, however, support may be requested or given in various ways.

1. No-strings contributions to departmental funds. This may mean single or recurrent payments, e.g. for a research fellow. These are difficult to stop.

2. Support to a department as a quid pro quo (e.g. for equipment).

3. Support of an individual as a quid pro quo (e.g. for travel to a congress). Any form of payment to subordinate staff without prior approval is wrong.

4. Support to an individual as a direct fee.

These call for care and discretion in ascending order. One has to keep an open mind and judge each situation on its merits. In practice the problem is not so difficult as it sounds because it seems to work out that the most mercenary of doctors are often least satisfactory investigators and they rapidly become known for what they are. By a process of natural selection, firms develop working relationships with certain doctors and departments with whom they get along well, and these can develop into a most fruitful and enjoyable partnership to which the firm should be able to contribute a good deal more than a few experimental compounds and some money.

All the same, there is no denying that there are difficult problems in this area. The timing of any payment is controversial. Some firms object to any advance agreement because it smacks of bargaining; others say that failure to agree beforehand too often leads to embarrassing misunderstandings.

There is no doubt about the need for general practitioner trials, but these are ethically and politically particularly delicate. They are often paid for on the basis of a fee for each case. Provided the first precept is scrupulously observed, payment for the work is justified. As always, so much depends on the individuals involved.

A particularly difficult problem is that academic and other departments often want continued support over a number of years but, in the present climate, any money that is available seems increasingly to be product-related and it is difficult to make long-term commitments even if a continued interest in a particular field seems likely. When practicable, a useful precaution and protection is to ensure that the panel of non-involved scientists previously referred to should also be informed of any money received.

It seems appropriate, as we are meeting in the Royal College of Physicians, to end with quotations from two of its Presidents. The first of these runs as follows: ' Certainly the greatest gap in the science of medicine is to be found in its final and supreme stage, the stage of therapeutics.' It was uttered by Sir Thomas Watson almost exactly one hundred years ago and he goes on: ' We want to learn distinctly what is the action of drugs . . . To me it has been a lifelong wonder how vaguely, how ignorantly, how rashly drugs are often prescribed.' (Watson, 1868). Of course, enormous strides have been made in the past 30 years, but they have in many respects only exaggerated the need for still better methods in drug evaluation. They have also increased the relevance of the second quotation from our distinguished President today, Sir Max Rosenheim, who said recently to the World Health Organization: ' I look forward to the great advances in knowledge that lie around the corner, but I do sometimes wonder whether the vast sums of money now being spent, in many countries, on research might not produce more rapid and spectacular improvement in world health if devoted to the application of what is already known.' (Rosenheim, 1968.)

REFERENCES

BINNS, T. B. & BUTTERFIELD, W. J. H. (1964). Clinical trials: Some constructive suggestions. *Lancet*, **1**, 1150.
BLOCH, H. & PAGET, G. E. (1968). Responsibilities of the pharmaceutical industry in the assessment of drug safety and efficacy. In *C.I.O.M.S. Round Table, Evaluation of Drugs: Whose Responsibility?* p. 47. Geneva: World Health Organization.
CAHAL, D. A. (1968). The role of regulatory agencies and industry in assessment of the safety of drugs for use in man: the situation in the United Kingdom. *Can. med. Ass. J.* **98**, 271.
GOLDBERG, L. (1965). The predictive value of animal toxicity studies carried out on new drugs. In *Clinical Testing of New Drugs*, p. 23. New York: Revere.
HILL, A. BRADFORD (1966). Reflections on the controlled trial. *Ann. rheum. Dis.* **25**, 107.
PAGET, G. E. (1965). Toxicity tests: a guide for clinicians. In *Clinical Testing of New Drugs*, p. 31. New York: Revere.
ROSENHEIM, M. (1968). Health in the world of tomorrow. *Lancet*, **2**, 821.
SPINKS, A. (1965). Justification of clinical trials of new drugs. In *Evaluation of New Drugs in Man*, Vol. 8, p. 7. Oxford: Pergamon.
WATSON, T. (1868). Present state of therapeutics. *Lancet*, **1**, 76.

THE PRACTICAL CONSIDERATIONS OF
SETTING UP A CLINICAL TRIAL

J. G. DOMENET

If clinical trials could always be conducted under ideal circumstances, much, if not all of this book, would become unnecessary. Indeed, clinical trials themselves would probably be superfluous, remaining as interesting academic exercises without which the true value of a drug would still be obvious. However, practical considerations impose limitations upon the design and execution of a trial and the ultimate success of the investigation is dependent on the trialist's ability to anticipate and cater for these practical difficulties.

Motivation

All trialists are human. This obvious fact introduces the first of many practical considerations which may affect the course of a clinical trial. A trialist may be motivated to undertake a study for one of many reasons and his ultimate aim may vary considerably. The motivation may be academic, an interest in the drug and its effect on the condition to be treated; financial, help towards the purchase of a piece of equipment for the department or a sponsored visit overseas; or self-advancement, material for a good publication.

Nowadays, the pharmaceutical firm manufacturing the drug to be studied is more than likely to have an interest in any trials involving it. Indeed, in the pre-marketing days of a compound, most trials will be instigated by the firm itself and even after marketing it will still seek to extend clinical investigations of the product.

The medical adviser to the pharmaceutical firm plays a vital role in the clinical investigation of its products and his overall knowledge of these drugs is second to none. It follows that any clinical trial will benefit from consultation with the relevant medical adviser who will provide not only his expert knowledge but also the firm's resources for the supply of active and placebo medication and the printing of all necessary documentation and record forms. The medical adviser is a specialist in the field of clinical trials and his services are free to the medical profession—' an opportunity not to be missed ', some might say.

Whatever the motivation for a clinical trial, one fact remains: all those involved must be satisfied with its design and execution. If not, this will be reflected in the way in which the study is conducted and bias may well be introduced, even subconsciously. To find, it is essential to look, and if one does not expect to find one may be tempted to look halfheartedly. This must be avoided and, therefore, the most important safeguard is in the careful preparation of the protocol.

The protocol

A successful trial is one which yields the correct answer to the question which was posed. It is entirely dependent on the validity of its protocol and should never be allowed to start until it is agreed that the protocol covers all foreseeable eventualities and ambiguities. To achieve this will almost certainly require several drafts and the cooperation of all concerned including statisticians, pharmacists, ward sisters and others. It cannot be too strongly stressed that time and effort expended at this stage will be amply rewarded later.

The format of the protocol will depend on individual taste. Whichever style is adopted, however, care should be taken that at least all the following points are considered and that the protocol is *written out in full.*

Object of the trial

In drawing up a protocol, it is wise to define firstly the object of the trial in simple terms. Though this may seem rather obvious, it is surprising how often one can ask this question of a ' trialist ' and receive the reply ' to see what happens, I suppose '. Whilst admitting that world shattering discoveries have been made by chance, Lady Luck is extremely busy and always grateful for a little help. In defining the object of a trial one ensures that everyone knows exactly the question which is to be answered and that what one is proposing to do is at all times relevant to the problem.

Rationale for the trial

It is a most useful exercise at this stage in the preparation of the protocol to set out the rationale for the proposed study. This requires that the relevant literature concerning the drug and that concerning the proposed indication be reviewed. It will then be seen whether the trial is intended to confirm previous findings, whether it is a logical progression on the basis of available evidence or whether a positive finding would be a ' long-shot '. It is evident that in the latter case much more stringent requirements will need to be met if the results are to be meaningful and acceptable.

Regulatory authorities

At this stage it is essential to check that the proposed study is within the area for which permission has been granted by the relevant official regulatory authority. In many countries, including the United Kingdom, it should be remembered that this permission applies not only to the drug itself but also to the indication for which it is to be used. Furthermore, these restrictions apply even when the trial is not organised by a pharmaceutical firm. If the trial is seen to fall outside the permitted area, permission must be sought. It may be helpful in this respect to present full details of the proposed study to the authority who may agree, under certain circumstances, to a single study without the need for a full submission of evidence.

Choice of trial design

There are certain practical considerations to be borne in mind when the choice of trial design is originally made. The most successful trial will be that which attempts not too little and not too much. The trial must be tailored to the facilities available and the temptation to stretch staff and equipment resisted. A well conducted open study, even without a comparative control, is better than a failed double-blind trial with multiple cross-overs. It must always be remembered, however, that a relatively simple trial can usually answer only relatively simple questions and care must be taken to ensure that the study being under-taken can answer the question being asked.

Most trials nowadays involve comparative controls, either active or placebo, and this may lead to some practical difficulties. It is usually essential that the study be blind but on occasion the formulations of the relevant active drugs are such that they cannot be presented in identical forms, and indeed, even the routes of administration may be different. In such cases, one can make use of the ' double-dummy ' technique which requires the manufacture of placebos for each of the active drugs. Patients may then be given both formulations at the same time, only one of which is placebo and the blind nature of the trial is maintained. For instance, in dealing with the problem of comparing the results of treating a skin condition topically with a cream or systemically with a tablet, both placebo cream and placebo tablets are prepared, each identical with the respective active prepara-tion. Patients selected for topical treatment will receive active cream and placebo tablets and vice-versa. This technique may be extended quite simply to more than two treatments, the limiting factors being the increasing opportunities for errors involved in dispensing and the numbers of tablets, capsules, suppositories, etc. which a patient is likely to be willing to take at any one time.

A variation on the double-dummy theme may be used when one wishes to compare a long-acting and a short-acting drug. In this case, placebos identical to the long-acting compound may be given as fre-quently as necessary to ensure that patients are receiving therapy with the same frequency whatever product is being administered. It is, of course, essential that the therapy is presented in such a way that the active long-acting medication is taken at the correct intervals and this can be achieved, for instance, by numbering the doses in the order in which they are to be taken. Needless to say, in order to maintain the blind nature of the trial, the short-acting drug is presented in a similar fashion even though all doses are active compound.

It is, of course, usual to ask for placebo medication to be identical with the active preparation but this is not always possible, and the

8

degree of match may vary from perfect to 'not very good'. Though a poor match is never to be encouraged, it is sometimes possible to accept something less than perfection. If the trial is so designed that the trialist or the patient will at some time be in possession or have access to both active and placebo medications at the same time, the degree of match necessary is such that it should be impossible to pick out either medication from a mixture of the two. If, however, active and placebo will only ever be handled separately, it is possible to allow a lesser degree of matching.

Criteria for inclusion of patients

Of paramount importance in the drawing up of the protocol will be the criteria which patients must meet to qualify for inclusion in the trial. Little difficulty should be encountered when these refer to objective parameters but a practical problem arises when selection involves a subjective assessment on the part of the trialist. If there is a possibility that more than one person may be entering patients into the trial independently, for instance a consultant and his registrar, a decision has to be taken whether a distinction will need to be made between these two groups. This problem of the comparability of patients is well recognised in multi-centre trials but it is not usually appreciated that it may occur in a single-centre trial. If the trial involves a surgical procedure it is essential that patients be matched according to the surgeon performing the operation. Indeed, consideration should also be given to the need to match for the anaesthetist.

The facilities available may also determine whether all patients meeting the criteria for inclusion will be entered into the trial or whether a selection will have to be made; for instance, the first two patients only at each clinic to be entered into the trial. This decision will be governed by such considerations as the laboratory facilities available for carrying out the required analyses, and the fact that follow-up attendances may be so spaced that cumulative interim totals may become impractical.

Criteria for exclusion of patients

The protocol must also define those patients who though meeting the criteria for inclusion, should be excluded for other reasons. These are usually related to co-existing diseases which form a contraindication to the drug under investigation or incompatibility of this drug with existing therapy which needs to be continued. Indeed, it is wise to specify in the protocol the contraindications to the drug and any precautions to be observed in its use. Known antidotes and methods of dealing with accidental overdosage should be detailed. Though one hopes that reference to these should not be necessary, their availability if required will be much appreciated.

Number of patients

The total number of patients who will be required to ensure a successful trial is of considerable practical importance. The statistician will usually have been able to indicate the theoretical number necessary to provide significant results on the basis of the type of trial being undertaken and the response rates anticipated. It may be found that the time required for this number of patients to be entered into the trial on the basis of, for example, incidence rates, would be such that it would be unlikely that continued interest in the study would be maintained or possibly that variations in other external factors might become significant. If this is so, it is imperative that the design be changed and an acceptable valid compromise agreed. It is difficult to be dogmatic about the total time which a trial should take from start to finish as this is very dependent on the actual study planned, but in the majority of cases, a year is more than enough.

Side-effects

The recording of side-effects is an essential part of any clinical trial and the method of doing so should be clearly stated in the protocol. In this connection, a number of practical considerations should always be borne in mind.

Firstly, a distinction should always be made between side-effects volunteered by the patient and those elicited by direct questioning. Where practicable, questioning with regard to side-effects should be withheld until the end of the trial, though this is obviously impossible in studies of long duration or in cross-over studies where the information would be required at each cross-over. When direct questioning is used, this should take the form of a pre-stated question put to all patients. ' Have the tablets disagreed with you in any way ' is a useful example.

Secondly, it is usually assumed that ' side-effects ' occurring during a trial are due to the medication. But these complaints may have been present before the trial started and it is recommended that in the initial assessment a question be put to each patient to determine what other complaints, if any, the patient has suffered from in the month preceding the start of the trial.

Methods and frequency of assessment

The success of the trial will depend on the validity and accuracy of the assessments made of each patient's progress. These in turn will depend on the competence of the staff and the availability of the necessary equipment and ancillary facilities. But even in the presence of competent staff and adequate facilities, failure may occur because of such factors as overloading. It may be wise in some instances to stagger entry of patients into a trial to ensure an even work load resulting from interim assessments during the course of the trial. In other cases, for instance where the major biochemical investigation requires 30 seconds to complete but the instrument needs calibrating before each period of use, it is more economical to ensure that as many investigations as possible are carried out at the one time. Holidays, for patients and staff, should not be overlooked. Most important of all is the fact that neither patients nor trialist be required to conform to a plan which will encourage them to default.

Drop-outs and defaulters

Rarely will a trial terminate without some patients dropping out or defaulting. This can be prevented to some extent by thoughtful design but many other factors cannot be overcome. Patients will move from the district, stop the trial because of side-effects or a feeling that they are not being helped or are cured, some will die. It is essential, therefore, that the protocol should clearly define in what way drop-outs and defaulters will be dealt with. It may be agreed that results available will be deleted or that they will stand but be analysed separately. Defaulting patients may need to be replaced by others. All these point must be clarified initially and careful instructions laid down as to procedures to be adopted.

Analysis of results

It is important to ensure that the correct results will be available to those carrying out the analysis at the right time and in the most convenient form. This latter consideration may dictate the format of the record cards which will usually be a compromise between the needs of the clinician and those of the statistician. It may be easier to analyse the results if they are presented in a certain order but this might not be the most logical one for the clinician to carry out his assessment. Since the statistician cannot produce the right results from incorrect data, it is obvious that, wherever necessary, the clinician's wishes should be given precedence.

In those trials where subsequent therapy depends on the interim analysis of results, care should be taken that such analysis is practical. Delays in the post, other commitments, holidays, etc. may well invalidate a perfectly reasonable ' plan '.

Mechanics of the trial

It is good practice to conclude the protocol with a section which details the practical steps to be followed during the trial. This can often be done by tracing a patient's course from initial assessment to the analysis of the results. By doing this, it is possible to see whether the various requirements and procedures outlined above are practical.

Likely sources of error or difficulty become obvious and may necessitate changes in the protocol or cautionary notices.

It is impossible to guarantee the smooth running of a clinical trial but there is no doubt that the careful preparation of a protocol covering all the factors mentioned above will improve the chances of success considerably.

THE MECHANICS OF THE CLINICAL TRIAL

A. W. GALBRAITH

The record form

When designed for a family doctor, the form should be brief and easy to complete. It is convenient if made to fit inside the National Health Service folder protruding half an inch at the top. The doctor is thus less likely to forget to fill in the form when the patient attends the surgery. A colour code can be useful if the doctor is carrying out more than one trial at a time. In Figure 1 is illustrated an elaborate form to be completed by a clinician with time at his disposal. The use of a special paper enables copies to be produced without the use of interleaved carbon. However the forms are particularly flimsy and each assessment requires a fresh top sheet. This sort of form could be used in hospital and should be designed to fit into the hospital notes. Most take A4 but some use quarto or even foolscap.

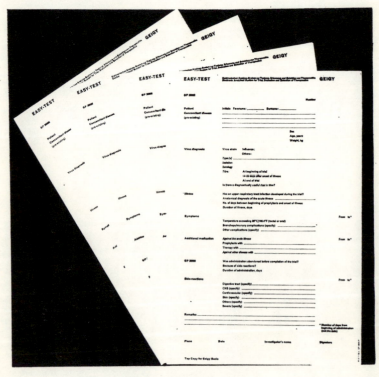

FIG. 1

Special clinical trial form.

To avoid having previous results in a rating scale available at subsequent interviews, the score is entered in the right hand column of a specially designed form. This column is torn from the form along a perforated line and stuck, for it has a gummed reverse surface, to a

EVENING OF DAY 1 (i.e. evening of the day you first saw the doctor)

How many tablets have you taken today?

Did the tablets disagree with you?   Yes / No

If so, in what way

Please think back to when you saw the doctor and try to compare the pain then with now.

Has the pain:— Quite gone
Still there, but less
Still there, but worse
About the same

If the pain is still there but less, can you say whether it is:— half gone   more than half gone   less than half gone. (Cross out those that do not apply)

If you think it will help to show how you feel, more clearly, try to fill in the blank square below. Pain is black, white is relief from pain and the four examples are given to help you. Compare the pain you have now with the pain when you saw your doctor.

  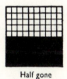 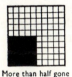   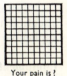

Pain   Half gone   More than half gone   Less than half gone   Your pain is?

EVENING OF DAY 2   Your name

Doctor's name

How many tablets have you taken today?

Did the tablets disagree with you?   Yes / No

If so, in what way

Please think back to THIS MORNING, and try to compare the pain now with then.

Has the pain:— Quite gone
Still there, but less
Still there, but worse
About the same

If the pain is still there but less, can you say whether it is:— half gone   more than half gone   less than half gone. (Cross out those that do not apply)

If you think it would help to show how you feel, more clearly, try to fill in the blank square below. Black represents pain, white relief from pain. Compare the pain you have now with that you had this morning.

    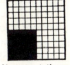   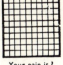

Pain   Half gone   More than half gone   Less than half gone   Your pain is?

FIG. 2

Form for the assessment of analgesia.

card which is filed separately. Subsequent interviews are recorded similarly.

Figure 2 is an example of what appears at first sight to be a simple method of assessing pain and its response to certain tablets. It proved a failure as the patients did not understand how to complete the blank square representing the amount of pain present or having disappeared.

It is a wise precaution to give a carbon copy of the proposed assessment form to the doctor and response sheets to a few typical patients, to see that they are entirely satisfactory, before going to the expense of printing special cards.

The use of different coloured cards can be useful. In one study, a green card recorded the patient's temperature, a red one the details relating to the index case, blue for the contacts and a yellow family record card. The simplicity of the design enabled the doctor to leave the cards in the patient's house and they were completed by a responsible adult. It is worthwhile to remember that often cards involve quite elaborate printing. The initial order will have to cover the typesetting and subsequent copies are relatively less expensive.

In summary, a record card should be designed with care and attention to detail. It is seldom possible to design a card which is applicable to more than one investigation.

Equipment

In many studies apparatus of varying complexity is required. For example, flow meters for a respiration study, exercise tolerance machinery for cardio-respiratory studies, grip-measuring gadgets for investigations in rheumatoid arthritis and laboratory equipment for biochemical estimations. Are these to be bought, borrowed, hired or donated? If different centres are pooling results, the apparatus must be standardised. One investigation was known to be nearly abandoned when the clinician noted three patients with an almost lethal acidosis which he attributed to the drug when in fact the pH meter was faulty.

Some trials involve intricate planning and this may be illustrated by reference to the investigation in general practice which utilised the coloured cards. A kit containing all the equipment necessary was posted to each family doctor taking part. Figure 3 shows the unavoidable bulk. Each box treats one family of up to six persons and each doctor considered that he might treat 10 families. In this study, a throat swab in transport medium for virus isolation was required and one wide-mouthed thermos flask was therefore given to each doctor.

Figure 4 illustrates the contents of each box, which included syrup and containers of the capsules under study, thermometer, response cards, syringes for venepuncture, elastoplast dressings, boxes to send the blood to the laboratory and envelopes to return the cards. The type of syringe used dispensed with the necessity of a separate container in that by removing the barrel when the syringe was full of blood and

THE MECHANICS OF THE CLINICAL TRIAL

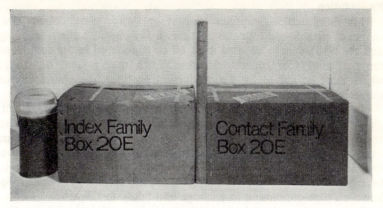

Fig. 3
Clinical trial kit.

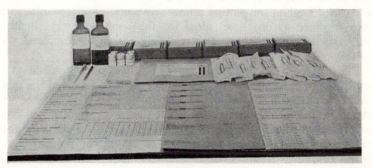

Fig. 4
Contents of kit.

replacing the needle by a blind hub, it formed a leak-proof container. To save the doctor having to write a label to stick on the blood specimen, each capsule container had a self-adhesive code-label top and bottom. The doctor peeled off the label on the bottom of the container and stuck it on to the first syringe container, the second blood specimen was labelled with the top label from the now empty capsule container. Each specimen was sent in a pre-paid addressed box to one laboratory where code numbers continued to be used and the serology was performed without any knowledge of the clinical situation. Incidentally, pre-paid labels have to be of a regulation size. An application is made to the General Post Office of the town receiving the mail for a registered number. Labels are then printed with the address together with this number, and money to cover the expected return deposited with the G.P.O.

Presentation

Matching tablets, capsules, creams or syrup; taste, colour, size, shape, consistency; disintegration time, assay check, coding, labelling and the containers to be used must all be considered in the context of the particular trial being undertaken. Each may present difficulties which must be solved by the production engineer, the pharmacist or the research department.

In the presentation of tablet or capsule medication to the patient, glass, plastic or aluminium containers are usually used. However, a small plastic bag can be useful for short runs where there is a change over of therapy or it is desired to increase the daily dosage by a specific amount. The name of the patient, code number and date to be taken can be written on the special matt surface. The bags are, however, time-consuming to package and fiddly to dispense.

Strip packing of tablets may be used in a clinical trial but this would probably involve a hand operated machine. It is advisable in such an instance for the individual responsible for the investigation to be present and supervise directly the packing procedure. This would be a useful method for putting up an active and an inert tablet to be taken together as one dose, ideal for the double-dummy situation. Time-consuming to prepare and relatively expensive compared with ordinary containers.

The use of a colour code may be used in the presentation of medication to the patient. As an example, one trial involved the treatment of pain in acutely ill patients, those less severely affected and patients suffering from chronic pain. The first group took tablets from boxes labelled in red, the second were in blue and the chronic group had green labelled boxes. The trial was in general practice but a clinical trial in a hospital usually involves the pharmacist. He can allocate active or placebo from code sheets upon receipt of specific information supplied by the clinician. If the pharmacist is to be involved, his advice and cooperation should be sought during the planning stage. If a consultant is seeing patients at different hospitals, it may be more convenient for him to be supplied with individual code-labelled containers. These should be carefully boxed so that the order of administration, if necessary, is obvious.

For the general practitioner, separate code-labelled containers are usually appropriate, but it should be noted at what intervals the patient is to be seen, the correct number of tablets or quantity of medicament supplied and the doctor instructed to collect the used container before issuing the next supply. When using a code, the key to each number may be held in a separate sealed envelope by each doctor in case of an emergency. In some cases it may be preferable for a neutral observer to hold the key.

As it is not unknown for non-production batches of matching tablets, syrups or creams to show unequal colour or consistency changes after a variable period of time, it is necessary to check the material from time to time otherwise the blind nature of the trial may be disturbed.

Follow-up

It is pointless to plan a regular assessment of any patient unless appointments are given and kept. The most valuable member of the team for this part of the exercise is the secretary. It may be necessary for the pharmaceutical firm concerned with the trial to supply part or full-time secretarial assistance. Printed appointment cards are useful to emphasise the importance of regular follow-up. Transport to the surgery may need to be provided for infirm or elderly patients. The services of a nurse or health visitor for domiciliary attendance can reduce the doctor's workload if the assessment can be carried out by such personnel. These apparently minor details may well make the difference between a steadily progressing trial and one which drifts on and on. Throughout the trial, the medical adviser, if he has been invited to participate, can be a useful link-man, chivvying the consultant, fortifying the family physician, pacifying the pharmacist, liaising with the laboratory or solacing the secretary.

STATISTICAL ANALYSIS OF CLINICAL TRIAL RESULTS

J. J. GRIMSHAW

Introduction

When the editors suggested the title of this paper, my first feeling was that the range was somewhat restrictive and that it would be difficult to gather enough material together. However, on trying to draft a framework I have been surprised to find the number of topics that could legitimately be included, and the problems have been entirely those of selection. I felt that it would not be appropriate to present a catalogue of statistical methodology, as the techniques referred to are described in a wide variety of statistical textbooks. Instead, I have tried to put together some thoughts on the analysis of clinical trials from the practical viewpoint, in order to illustrate some of the problems that arise in this phase of the work, and to show you the type of approach that a statistician uses.

Design and analysis

Earlier papers have already dealt with the design stage of a clinical trial but it is important to remember that the dichotomy into design and analysis—adopted for this symposium—is rather artificial. To a great extent the limitations to the analyses available to you are imposed by decisions made at the design stage, and it is at this stage that the nature of the analysis to be finally performed should be discussed. It is the design that defines the analysis and it is the proposed analysis that should define the method of recording the data.

During analysis it is almost inevitable that some flaws in design will emerge and although some of these can be corrected retrospectively, frequently all one can do is to note the points emerging and remember them in subsequent trials. If one wished to use an ' in ' expression for this technique, I suppose it could be called *sequential feedback*.

Since flow charts are popular, this is simply illustrated in Figure 1. Because statisticians are supposed to deal in probabilities I have allocated 20 per cent of all necessary modifications to an editorial monitoring of the records from a current trial. For the other 80 per cent of changes you can only modify future trials.

The most important arrow in the network is the dangling 80 per cent at the end. I sometimes think we never learn from our mistakes. Although I have been associated with clinical trials, in one way or another, for just over sixteen years, I have never yet studied the final records without wishing changes had been made either in what was collected or the way it was recorded.

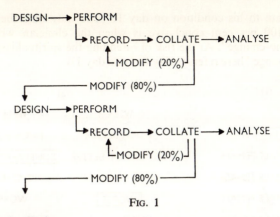

FIG. 1

Editing and collating

This inevitably leads on to the problems of editing and collating. You may be wondering what all this has to do with the statistical analysis of results. The answer is that the practice of medicine is rapidly changing. The clinician of today has been dragged, protesting loudly, to the very brink of numeracy: he is replacing some of the old subjective mumbo-jumbo by an objective set of data supported by clear statements pertaining to probabilities, significance, error and so on. To this end we all spend a great deal of time on randomisation, pairing of patients and other procedures designed to remove bias; and yet the bias introduced by the need to edit badly designed record cards goes a long way to explain some of the discrepancies between and within trials.

It is incredibly difficult to design a card that will not give rise to some problems at the analysis stage and I would like to give you three simple examples of the sort of problem the statistician is faced with. The first example (Figure 2) concerns the sex of the patient. What is the sex of the five patients (a) to (e)? The first one is obvious—'ringing' an alternative is the one clear unambiguous response. So too is (b)—we can accept that if one alternative is firmly crossed out, the other is the required response; (c) is for clinicians who are introverted and negativistic and (d) is for the extrovert. All these answers so far say 'male', but what about (e)? On the whole I would read this as 'male'—one can imagine someone filling in the form and saying 'sex'?—oh yes 'male', but I was severely shaken half-way through an analgesic test, when some years ago one of these 'males' was said to have dysmenorrhoea.

The second example is very common. Response (often pain) is assessed by the patient at weekly intervals. At the end of week 1 this particular patient was worse than when he started; but what does 'some improvement' mean in week 2? Has his 'worse' state improved to what he was at the beginning of the trial or does 'some improvement' relate to his condition on day 1? (The only time the referring point is 100 per cent conclusive is when the clinician writes ' ill ', ' dead ', ' no-change '. At the risk of offending the spiritualists, I reckon the ' no-change ' here refers to day 8 not to day 1!)

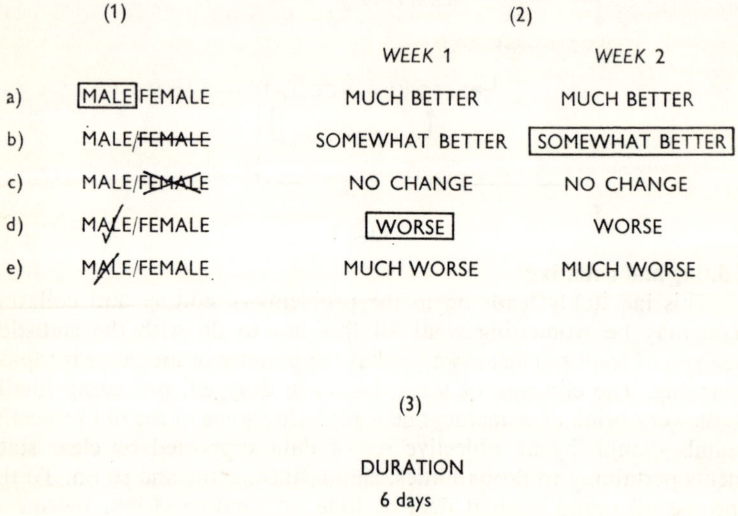

	(1)		(2)
		WEEK 1	WEEK 2
a)	MALE FEMALE	MUCH BETTER	MUCH BETTER
b)	MALE/FEMALE	SOMEWHAT BETTER	SOMEWHAT BETTER
c)	MALE/FEMALE	NO CHANGE	NO CHANGE
d)	MALE/FEMALE	WORSE	WORSE
e)	MALE/FEMALE	MUCH WORSE	MUCH WORSE

(3)

DURATION
6 days

SO YOU THINK YOU CAN DESIGN A RECORD CARD?
FIG. 2

The last example is trivial, but again, often occurs. Does ' duration ' refer to dosing, illness since dosing began, or total duration of illness including any pre-dosage period? Any of these three measurements could be called ' duration ' and I have seen all three used by different clinicians in the same trial. Indeed, one often meets the situation in analysing trials data where it becomes clear that one clinician has placed one interpretation on such a question as the last whereas other clinicians have put other interpretations. Occasionally it is possible to go back to the clinician concerned in cases of doubt but quite often one can only either make an inspired guess or leave the response out altogether.

In multi-centre trials, variations in interpretation are particularly common; so too are variations in the standard of filling in the pro formas. A commonly occurring situation is where responses from one centre seem to be out of line with those from all other centres. Sometimes, there may be good reasons for this, perhaps unforeseen. The higher proportion of fried foods in the diet of Midland industrial town dwellers compared with rural workers in the South of England may modify drug adsorption patterns and, for example, reduce the incidence of G.I. side effects. If such a difference is found, however, the more common explanation is that in one particular centre side effects were not specifically enquired about. This is a mistake that is difficult to right retrospectively—people's memories are rarely to be trusted—but in a future trial one would modify the record card to read '*volunteered* side effects' and 'if none volunteered ask about G.I. —— etc.' It is important to realise, when we come to the collation stage, that 'no entry' is not always equivalent to zero-response: it may mean 'not asked', 'not relevant at this centre' or even 'I forgot to fill it in'.

The question of who should do the editing of the data is a vexed one. I take the view that if the card has been properly designed this work is best done by the statistician. I would not claim that he would always make the correct data editing decision if he is medically untrained but he will always try to apply an unbiased judgement. I would like to give one example of this problem. In a recent antibiotic trial, the progress of several presenting symptoms was assessed at intervals. Some doctors participating filled in 'marked improvement' in the clinical response section when all presenting symptoms had improved but not all had completely resolved. A few wrote 'cured' against this category. On statistical analysis I took the first more stringent definition of 'cure' but the clinician who set up the trial disagreed. 'Ah yes," he said 'but it is well known, for example, that swollen glands can persist for weeks and we would be justified in claiming a cure for these cases'. Now, I don't for a moment question his judgement, but this raises one or two interesting points.

1. If this was a truly unbiased comment—and I am sure it was—it should have been considered at the design stage and the card produced accordingly. A full definition of 'cured' *v* 'improvement' should have been given to the participating doctors and to the statistician.

2. Suppose that two drugs 'E' and 'P' produced exactly the same 'cure' rate on the modified definition. We would be quite justified in terming the drugs equi-active. Now suppose that for drug 'P'—for some reason or other—the patients glands had regressed (whereas on 'E' they had not) what do we say now?

Have we a super cure category? Have we got the classic case of two equal drugs with one being more equal than the other? Would we perhaps comment on this if 'P' was our drug but dismiss it as misleading and irrelevant if it belonged to a competitor? My only plea is, if a clinician is to do the editing before the data are statistically analysed, let him be quite sure that when he says 'Ah yes, what Dr X meant was so-and-so', he shouldn't really be saying 'What I would have liked Dr X to have meant is so-and-so'.

I have spent a long time on this section because although the editing and collation of data is an integral part of the analysis, it is rarely mentioned in clinical trial discussions.

I will say once again: there is more error and bias unwittingly introduced into clinical trials at the data editing stage, than from any other single factor in the procedure.

Scales of measurement and the analytical model

Let us assume that you have cleared the hurdle of editing, you have coded the data, you have tabulated in a series of two-way tables and added up rows and columns. Finally you have looked at each other in horror and said ' This will never convince The Committee on Safety of Drugs, I suppose we'll have to let the statistician see it '.

The first thing a statistician will do is to check all the arithmetic, because just as every clinician has profound contempt for the clinical acumen of his statistical colleague, so no statistician will ever believe that a clinician can add up a column of figures.

Then he will sit down and carefully check the quality of each section of the data for this will define the range of permissible analysis. In this sense ' quality ' has a special connotation.

Typical clinical trials data can be conveniently divided into four scale categories:

1. Purely qualitative, head counting data. Classification with no conceivable scalar properties.

2. (At the other end of the scale) data which have a logical numerical internal relationship and which can be handled by a selection of powerful analytical tools.

3. Data, which although numerical in the above sense, are better dealt with by qualitative methods.

4. (The corollary to 3) Data which although strictly qualitative we would like to regard as quantitative—an end often achieved by applying some sort of scale, sometimes bogus.

For the purpose of this exercise, let us consider data from a hypothetical, but fairly typical trial; we will imagine that each of two groups of 50 chronic bronchitics have been randomly allocated to one of two presumed active drugs and studied over a fixed period—say three weeks dosage. Although double-blind and randomised, the trial was not a cross-over, so the between drug difference is a clear cut comparison between the responses of the two groups of patients. Many facts will have been recorded during the trial, but I want to concentrate on just four of them: Age, Sex, FEV (measured on day 1 and again on day 20) and overall assessment of response at the end of treatment (classed as marked improvement, some improvement, no change, worse, much worse).

Sex (variate type 1). Although I suppose to be fashionable, one should regard sex as a continuum on a scale ranging from -1 to $+1$, from the practical point of view it is a purely classificatory variable. One writes ' male ' or ' female ' and this fully defines our variable.

Each group of patients will have its own sex ratio and together with age distribution one can form the traditional two-way table comparing the age and sex distribution of the two groups.

TABLE I

Age	Group I		Group II	
	Male	Female	Male	Female
20-29				6
30-39	1		2	
40-49	5	1	6	1
50-59	29	2	19	1
60-69	9		13	1
70-	3		1	
Total	47	3	41	9

Having produced the table (Table I) the next step is to analyse the results and we have three questions to answer as far as sex is concerned: (1) Is there a different sex ratio between the two groups? (2) Is the difference statistically significant and/or meaningful? (3) If it is what are we going to do about it?

Well, the first answer is obvious. The proportion of females in Group 1 is 0·06 and in Group 2 it is 0·18, so there is certainly a difference.

For testing the statistical significance of the difference we can use any of the methods available for qualitative data. With cell frequencies of this size one could, for example, form the familiar 2x2 contingency table and calculate a χ^2 based on 1 degree of freedom (Table II).

TABLE II

	Male		Female		Total
	O	E	O	E	
Group I	47	44	3	6	50
Group II	41	44	9	6	50
Total	88	88	12	12	100

$$\chi^2 = 3\cdot41 \ (\chi^2 \text{ for } P = 0\cdot05 = 3\cdot84)$$

Alternatively, one could use the more generalised formula for testing differences between two proportions (Fig. 3).

9

GROUP I   MALES 47 (p_1=0.94 q_1=0.06)

GROUP II   MALES 41(p_2=0.82 q_2=0.18)

$p_1 - p_2$=0.12, STANDARD ERROR

$$\text{OF DIFFERENCE} = \sqrt{\frac{p_1 q_1}{nl} + \frac{p_2 q_2}{n2}} = 0.0639$$

$$z = 1.88 \quad (P = 0.06)$$

Fig. 3

By either test we look up the appropriate table of probabilities and find P just greater than 0·05 by the χ^2 test and 0·06 by the exact test. Either way we have an answer that is just outside the frequently chosen level of statistical significance. We could, therefore, salve our consciences by saying ' Yes, there is a difference in sex ratio, but it is not statistically significant therefore we can ignore it '. However : —

1. The level of 5 per cent is a purely arbitrary ' action level '. There are many occasions when we should take action on a much lower level of significance perhaps 10 per cent or even lower.

2. A difference at the magnitude found should always make us think twice—never mind the statistical significance. It is almost certainly meaningful.

As far as the third question is concerned (What do we do about it?) the answer is fairly obvious in this case. We would look with grave suspicion at the 6 females aged 20 to 29 in Group 2 (remembering that they are supposed to be chronic bronchitics) and we would check on the criteria for admission to the trial to make quite sure that patients suffering from an aftermath of Asian Flu—or whatever—haven't been included by mistake.

A more difficult question to answer is ' to what extent is my sample representative of the whole population of chronic bronchitis '? and hence ' how good is the predictive capacity of this trial?' This leads me into a plea for a more intelligent use of demographic data than is generally made in the analysis of trial results. In this respect I think that the statistician is more culpable than the clinician but I will return to this point later.

FEV (*variate type 2*). This is an example of a typical quantitative variable and many techniques are open to us. We can consider several sources of variation at once and perform an analysis of variance; we can derive individual means with their associated standard errors and perform a series of ' t ' tests; we can rank the improvements noted and carry out a non-parametric test of some description; or we could even reduce the data still more by assigning some notional degree of improvement as ' effective ' and any less improvement as ' non-effective ', thus partitioning the data for each drug into two classes, and then perform a χ^2 test as described in the last section. Broadly speaking, the above methods are in descending order of sophistication and furthermore, they make decreasing demands of our knowledge of the distribution underlying the measurement of FEV.

We have to steer a course between throwing away a lot of information and presenting an over elaborate analysis—which helps no one.

The important criterion is that in the trial under discussion, we are trying to discriminate between the responses in two groups of patients Drug A and Drug B. Which method of analysis we use depends to a large extent on the magnitude of the expected effect.

Consider, for example, the situation in the treatment of bronchospasm, if isoprenaline was not generally available. Suppose the drug was given to you and you tested it in one group of patients, against a placebo inhaler in the other. There is no doubt at all that a simple partition into ' effective ', ' non-effective ' would soon show up isoprenaline as an active drug. Indeed, in any trial involving a test of active drug against placebo, I would want to be able to show an effect by a simple classificatory test of this kind. As your test drugs become more alike in response, so you have to use more sophisticated statistical methods to show the *statistical* significance of an observed mean difference in effect, but this is *all* you do. *Nothing, but nothing will alter the clinical significance of your observed difference.* All the statistician can do is to remove all the assignable causes of variation so that you can compare the difference with a residual random error. If this finally tells you that the mean increase in FEV for drug A is 50 ml greater than for drug B, and that this difference is very highly significant, well good-oh! for statistics—it is up to you to justify the significance clinically.

Without going into the algebra, what are the sources of variation we would look for in this situation? How would we attempt to allow for them?

1. Firstly we would—at any one time—perform three tests in sequence and the residual ' within patient—within day ' error would be our basic estimate of error variance.

2. Secondly, we would say that a patient's FEV varies widely from day to day and a single measurement at Day 1 followed by another at Day 20 is unrealistic—so we would in practice take measurement on several different days throughout the trial and look for the trend.

3. Thirdly, we might perhaps ask if the response we are measuring is universally relevant. For example, if we are testing a broncholytic, is there perhaps a maximum value to the FEV, above which we would classify the patient as not suffering from bronchospasm, and hence not to be included in the analysis? If there is such a notional maximum, does it vary from patient to patient, and if so how do we define it?

4. Fourthly, my deliberate mistake. The astute amongst you have

already said 'Ah, but we wouldn't do a trial like that in any case. Every first year medical student knows that all trials should be cross-over. We would test both drugs in each patient and compare his response'.

Well, this is fine in theory, and there are many occasions when a cross-over trial is of real value. Generally what happens when you come to analyse the results is that—with the best will in the world—you would find that 58 patients started on drug A and 42 on drug B: and for any situation where some depressed value is returning to normal after drug treatment, there is inevitably a pronounced order effect. In the usual situation where you have an imbalance in numbers of the sort I have described, you can no longer separate a possible gain in response to drug A, from the fact that more patients started on drug A than B.

The way out of this one if you want to use a cross-over design is to use two or more exacerbations of bronchitis in the same patient and to test A on one occasion and B on another. In any case you only gain on using the within patient variance, if the difference between the patients is large; e.g. consider a cross-over design of two drugs on 50 patients and suppose each drug is assessed once (Table III):

TABLE III

Source	df	MS
Between drugs	1	A
Between patients	49	B
Residual	49	C
Total	99	

In the cross-over (or paired) test you are comparing, as an F ratio, A/C. However, if you have the situation where the difference between patients is small compared with the error of measurement, a more sensitive test is obtained by pooling B and C and comparing A with an error mean square based on 98 degrees of freedom. This is exactly equivalent to the unpaired case.

So, in summary, the cross-over design is not always appropriate, and even if it is, it doesn't necessarily follow that you have a gain in sensitivity.

5. Finally, there is one other method of reducing error variance that I must mention, and that is the use of concomitant information. The actual algebra at the analysis of variance stage gets a little bit hairy, but in essence the basic principles are simple. Taking as an example the trial we are discussing, let us suppose that within a block of patients—all treated with one drug—we plot response against initial

FEV value and find a relationship; for example, we might find a high response at a low initial FEV value, but a decreasing response at higher initial values.

Let us suppose that this relationship exists for two drugs which are equally effective in action, but that the mean initial FEV for the two groups are different. (1·0L for Drug A, 1·5L for Drug B).

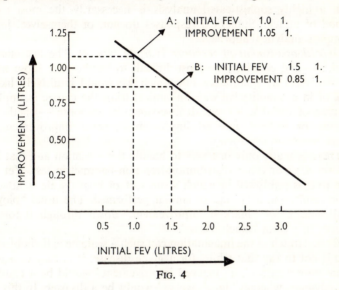

FIG. 4

As Figure 4 shows you will now have an apparent but meaningless difference in favour of drug A.

The analysis of co-variance technique corrects for this by adjusting the observed responses to allow for differences in the starting means.

Although the principles of this technique are fairly easy to grasp—in practice it is rather complicated to apply, for even if the response in one group of patients can be shown to be related to the initial value, it does not follow that this exact relationship holds for the other drug.

Even more complicated is the fact that the dependence is frequently non-linear. The response of a patient with bronchospasm to isoprenaline—for example—shows a pronounced optimum round about an initial FEV of 1·5L, but this response falls off rapidly on each side of this initial value. Nevertheless, the use of concomitant variables of this sort can occasionally substantially reduce the bias as well as the residual error of trial.

Age (variate type 3). At first sight, age is a typical quantitative variable, and one can indeed derive a mean and standard error, and perform ' t ' tests etc. In practice though, we are interested in the pattern of age distribution for each drug and possibly for each sex within each drug group. Furthermore, if we wish to make valid predictions about the use of the drug in the whole population of patients suffering from the disease, it is really incumbent upon us to show that our sample is representative of the parent population. For these purposes I have generally found that a qualitative assessment—of the χ^2 type— is more informative than the traditional ' t ' test approach. In other words, it doesn't follow that because the data exists in a quantitative form, a highly sophisticated analysis is necessarily the most useful method of attack. Numerical responses do not, of themselves, justify a complex analytical approach.

Overall assessment of response (variate type 4). The last class of variables—and certainly the most difficult to handle—are those which are unmistakably qualitative but which we would intuitively like to think of in a quantitative way. In clinical trials the classic example of this type of variable is ' overall assessment of response '—whether by clinician or patient (marked improvement, some improvement, no change, worse, much worse).

There is really only one way to handle this situation and that is to perform a χ^2 or other distribution-free non-parametric test. Yet trial after trial is published in which some sort of bogus scale is attached to the result, and a ' t ' test or similar performed. The usual ' ploy ' is to allocate 2 for ' marked improvement ' down through 0 for ' no change ' to −2 for ' much worse '.

By no stretch of the imagination can such a scale be called objective. Who is not to say that while, for a given disease, it is easy to achieve ' some improvement ', a ' marked improvement ' would be a considerable advance, whereas ' much worse ' would be a disaster. In this case it may be more realistic to score 10, 1, 0, −10, −20. In other words, we cannot assume linearity over our classification scale.

For an objective measurement such as FEV, the mean value has reality—it is possible to imagine a patient with precisely this value— indeed, if we make many measurements it will occur frequently for several patients. But what on earth does a mean score of 0·75 on the clinical response scale imply? That we are three-quarters of the way from ' no change ' to ' some improvement '?

As an example consider the following possible outcome of the trial we have been looking at (Table IV). On drug B, four patients are somewhat worse—which is a poor outcome, 20 have shown a substantial improvement which is excellent, and 22 have shown no change at all. On drug A, 38 patients have improved to some extent (18 marked improvement), and only 4 have shown no change, but 8 are much worse which is serious. Statistics will soon show you that the difference between the classifications is significant. (In this case $\chi^2 = 21·93$, $P < 0·001$.) However this does not tell you which drug is the *better*. It is up to *you* as clinicians to say whether the gain in overall improvement for drug A is more important than the fact that very poor responses were obtained in 8 patients.

TABLE IV

	Scale I	Scale II	Drug A	Drug B
Marked improvement	2	10	18	20
Some improvement	1	1	20	4
No change	0	0	4	22
Worse	−1	−10	—	4
Much worse	−2	−20	8	—
Total score (Scale I)			40	40
Mean score (Scale I)			0·80	0·80
Total score (Scale II)			40	164
Mean score (Scale II)			0·80	3·28

If you try and fit ' scores ' to tell you which is the better drug, you will immediately see the fallacy, for on scale I (2, 1, 0, −1, −2) the mean score is 0·8 for each drug, whereas on scale II (10, 1, 0, −10, −20) the mean score is 0·8 on drug A but 3·28 on drug B; and you can obtain any other balance of scores you like by adjusting the scale accordingly.

The *decisions* that you make following the analysis of data from a trial are no more valid than the data themselves warrant. It sometimes seems to me that some clinicians—none of course present today—use statistics as a drunk uses a lamp-post—for support rather than illumination.

Use of demographic data

I mentioned earlier the need to show the predictive power of what is often a restricted clinical trial in terms of the total population of patients suffering from the disease. Much published information is available from the Ministry of Health, the Registrar General's Office, the Office of Health Economics and numerous other official sources. There is also available data from one's own previous clinical trials in the field, and, from publications from collaborators and, indeed, competitors. Ideally, this information should be available for every disease category in which the company is interested. The impetus for collecting the data should come from the clinical research department but the task falls squarely on the shoulders of the statistics/market research departments.

Differences in response may well be related to physical location, ethnic differences, social class, dietary habits and a host of other factors—genetic, social, and environmental. In general far too little use is made of the wealth of information available, which might well broaden the base of a trial.

Single drug trial

This situation is particularly apparent in the case of the single drug trial. In a single drug trial, you are acquiring ' safety in use ' data in large numbers of patients. Traditionally the drug is farmed out to a wide range of G.P.'s—across the country—to be tried in every case that appears relevant. What a wonderful opportunity to study just those factors that I have described and, their interactions on each other! In the traditional comparative clinical trial, we are essentially interested in the mean response of two (or more) groups of patients. The question we are asking is ' Is drug A better than drug B?' We are only interested in the ' forest ', there isn't time to look at the trees. In the single drug trial, we *are* interested in the trees. Why does a beech at Andover flourish, but an ash at Basingstoke wither and rot? I know that, in general, the Committee on Safety of Drugs prefer controlled trials, but I cannot believe that a trial of the sort I have described, which was properly documented and added something to our knowledge of the protean effects of our drug, would not be welcomed. There is a very real place for a single drug trial, if only to give us time to stop and think.

Combining results

A few words on combining results from several trials, a subject I touched on briefly when discussing editing multi-centre data.

We come up against stark reality when two consecutive trials of A against B are analysed. In one A is significantly better than B: in the second B is significantly better than A. What do we do? What does it mean?

Within one company what we should do is quite easy to define. We should *critically* examine five factors in the trial.

1. The criterion for admission
2. the *gross* comparability of patients
3. the dosage schedule, including dosing in relation to body weight, and total duration of dosage
4. the record card and our instructions to clinicians and to patients
5. the scoring system—if one was used—and the method of analysis.

If all these factors are really identical, it means that there is some other factor affecting response that we have failed to take into account and, if necessary retrospectively, we should try and extract some of the data of the type that have been described earlier.

If Company Y publishes the results on Drug A, and Company Z publishes the other set, the situation is rather different. I would have thought that it was of benefit to both companies to get at the truth, and a collaborative investigation along the lines I have suggested should be set up by the clinicians concerned getting together—if necessary with the statisticians.

If we wish to pool data from several consecutive trials on our own drug, the same careful matching is necessary. If the trials are spread over a long period differences in seasonality must be considered, both in terms of incidence of a disease and possibly also its response to a given drug. All the criteria for matching apply and if different doses of drug have been used or different comparative drugs employed, this is really a rather difficult situation. I can add together 1 lb of apples and $1\frac{1}{2}$ lb of pears and easily work out a mean weight of a single 'fruit'— but what the definition of 'fruit' is in terms of the original apple or pear, is anyone's guess.

What I have tried to do in this paper is to illustrate some of the problem areas in the analysis of clinical trials—particularly those areas which are seldom discussed. As a last thought to leave you with I must emphasise once again that all the statistician can do is to make allowance for assignable causes of variation and hence present the analysis in such a way that it will aid your decision. The responsibility for assigning *clinical* significance is yours and yours alone.

Statisticians can do many things, but they cannot work miracles— that is your job!

THE CLINICIAN'S INTERPRETATION OF TRIAL RESULTS

E. L. HARRIS and J. D. FITZGERALD

Hill (1960) said '. . . to be fruitful, I believe that, without pretending to expert knowledge, the clinician must think statistically and the statistician must think clinically. Only by so doing, can the statistician learn what is useful, and what is useless, to bring into his counting machine; only thus can the clinician learn the importance of experimental design and the precision required of him.' The final purpose in evaluating the effects of a new therapy is to demonstrate its absolute and relative efficacy and safety. Because clinical trials are biological experiments carried out in heterogenous material capable of considerable natural variation, most of the measurements of effect must be analysed statistically. The clinician, when reading reports of such studies, is immediately faced with the problem of distinguishing results which demonstrate a statistically significant difference in response, between a control and a treated group, from results which are of clinical importance—or significance.

In the clinical context, the word significant implies that what is observed is notable, or important, or worthy of consideration. In the statistical sense, it implies that the mean results in comparing two or more groups, differ from each other by more than twice the standard error. It is known that such a difference could occur by chance relatively rarely (normally 5 times in 100 tests), and, therefore, the difference in results is said to be ' significant '. The criterion of ' significance ' can be altered so that whilst for most purposes twice the standard error is used, the level can be raised to three times the standard error when the difference would occur by *chance* only once in 370 tests. Statistical significance gives a measure of the probability of the observed difference being real, rather than occurring by chance. It implies also that when random samples are taken from one of the groups under study, there will not be a ' significant ' difference between them. It must be borne in mind that when ' no significant difference ' is said to be present between two groups, it means rather that the difference is *not proven,* rather than that there is a proven lack of difference.

The readers of clinical trials reports can be misled in two ways. Firstly, they may conclude from an article which shows a statistically significant effect in favour of a new therapy, that a clinically significant effect will be observed if the therapy is used in their own patients (Type A error). Secondly, they may conclude that because there was no statistical difference in response between a control and a treated group, that the treatment will be of no value in any patient (Type B error).

Many sources of error and misinterpretation can arise. A common one arises in the conversion of clinical observations or criteria into mathematical terms for the purpose of statistical analysis. For example, in a double blind trial of the therapy of post operative abdominal distension, the chief criterion was the degree of distension of the abdomen under two treatment regimes, administered on a double blind basis. The distension was reported as $+$, $++$, $+++$, or $++++$. The actual measurement was carried out by abdominal palpation, which even in experienced hands, can only gauge differences in distension very roughly. Yet the results were given sophisticated statistical analysis and statistically significant differences were demonstrated between the treatment and placebo (Type A error).

Another manoeuvre is to give an arbitrary weighting to a constellation of symptoms, and then determine the effects of treatment on these symptoms. This type of analysis has been used successfully by Wayne for the clinical evaluation of thyrotoxicosis. The method was very carefully validated before being offered for general clinical use. A recent report of an anti-anginal drug trial, however, used a weighting scale to take into account mild, moderate, and severe attacks of angina. But nowhere in the paper was it laid down what constitutes the difference between a mild and severe attack of angina. Is it the amount of discomfort the patient feels? This is impossible to assess. Is it the duration of the attack of pain? If so, then it must be related to the precipitating factor, because a patient can alter a mild attack to a severe one by continuing to exercise for some urgent reason. The results of this trial were given a most thorough statistical analysis, but it was impossible to gauge the quality of the fundamental observations. In general, therefore, one must scrutinize the validity of the clinical observations, and ensure that the correct criteria in relation to the desired result are selected for statistical analysis.

The way in which fallacious criteria of response can mislead the statistician into drawing fallacious conclusions about a drug's therapeutic place can be seen by an analysis of another trial of an anti-anginal agent, This multi-centre trial, concerning 350 patients, was a double-blind, randomised, crossover study, comparing the anti-anginal agent and its placebo. Each patient was treated for periods of eight weeks with each medication, and when all the results were analysed, the computer into which these had been fed churned out the result that the experimental drug was significantly better than placebo.

However, on reading the methodology more closely it appeared that this conclusion was based on some very dubious clinical criteria of response. These were:

1. There were 30 per cent fewer attacks of anginal pain in one period compared with the other.

2. A 30 per cent reduction in glyceryl trinitrate tablet intake.

3. A negative Master ' 2-step ' test after active drug coupled with a positive response after placebo.

4. Improvement in exercise tolerance as judged by the patient.

5. Improvement in dyspnoea—patient's assessment.

6. Overall feeling of well being.

The most important criterion of response to a prophylactic anti-anginal agent is a reduction in the frequency of attacks. This may be coupled with a reduction in the consumption of glyceryl trinitrate tablets as a confirmatory index. Re-analysis of the trial findings showed that on this criterion there was no difference between ' active ' drug and placebo. The statistician, however, not realising the relative importance of the various criteria, combined all of these in an ' all factors satisfactory ' analysis and came to the conclusion that the test drug was significantly better than placebo; a conclusion which from the clinical point of view is not valid (Type A error).

This particular trial also demonstrated another of the many pitfalls for the uninitiated. One of the criteria employed to assess response was the standard Master ' 2-step ' exercise test. The clinician carrying out the study did not take into account the physiological changes in circulation which occur after exercise, for it has been demonstrated that exercise tolerance improves following exercise and that this improvement may persist for periods up to 30 minutes after such exercise. In this particular study the average time interval between the control period and the drug period of exercise was 12 minutes whereas with placebo it was 45 minutes. This discrepancy clearly invalidates the findings from the test as used in this trial, and demonstrates the need for careful clinical appraisal of trial methodology.

To turn to another important role of the clinician when assessing clinical trial reports, one must consider in some detail the term ' clinical significance '. This has been defined as the *value* which the prescribing physician puts to a therapy (Maxwell, 1968). This can be looked at in several ways, possibly the most important is the danger of a satisfactory response in a small number of patients being swamped by an overwhelming failure rate in the majority. The difference in response could possibly be accounted for by a genetically determined, low incidence, metabolic anomaly.

The frequency distribution curve (number of persons showing a particular response plotted against the magnitude of response) is usually Gaussian in character, but in one or two instances the distribution curve shows two distinct peaks demonstrating the presence of two different types of individuals and, therefore, two different types of genes in the population (Crampton and Pride, 1966). A good example is those individuals who have an abnormal pseudocholinesterase because they will continue to respond to the muscle relaxant succinylcholine for periods of up to 30 to 50 minutes whereas the majority of subjects respond for only 2 to 4 minutes.

A further instance is the occurrence of slow and fast acetylators of isoniazid. The slow acetylators require a much smaller dose and when given the normal dose are likely to suffer from nerve damage. Thus, in every trial, the overall response of each individual patient should be carefully examined in order to avoid a type B error.

The problem is that potentially useful drugs for minority group patients may be lost to therapeutics. This will become less important as knowledge of biological typing increases. At present many trial reports do not even contain details of the criteria laid down in the protocol for patient selection.

Another aspect of clinical significance hinges on what is defined as an acceptable level of response. In the example of the anti-anginal drug trial, one of the criteria of response was a 30 per cent reduction in attacks of anginal pain. This is a very arbitrary figure and a level of 25 per cent could have been selected, and some patients would be grateful for even a 10 per cent reduction in frequency of attacks.

If there is a lesson that can be learnt from this it is that every doctor must look very critically at clinical trial reports and must apply his own clinical experience to the trial protocol, criteria of response and other parameters employed. But with increasing specialisation and the ever-increasing volume of clinical trials reports, it becomes virtually impossible for the average doctor to review critically each study. He therefore must rely to some extent on the standards imposed by the editorial policy of the journal in which the report is printed. A heavy responsibility thus falls on editors especially if the present standard of clinical trial design and reporting is to be improved. The danger is that editors may swing too far allowing a blind acceptance of double blind trials without a critical evaluation of their shortcomings and their ability to mislead as well as to lead (Cromie, 1963).

REFERENCES

CRAMPTON, R. F. & PRIDE, E. (1966). Factors affecting and methods for assessing dosage. In *Symposium on The Dosage of Medicines*, p. 3. London: The Pharmaceutical Society of Great Britain.
CROMIE, B. W. (1963). The feet of clay of the double-blind trial. *Lancet*, **2**, 994.
HILL, A. BRADFORD (1960). Aims and ethics. In *Controlled Clinical Trials*, p. 7. Oxford: Blackwell.
MASTER, A. M. & ROSENFELD, I. (1961). The 'two-step' exercise test brought up to date. *N.Y. St. J. Med.* **61**, 1850.
MASTER, A. M. & ROSENFELD, I. (1961). Criteria for the clinical application of the 'two-step' exercise test: Obviation of false-negative and false-positive responses. *J. Amer. med. Ass.* **178**, 283.
MAXWELL, C. (1968). The significance of significance. *Clin. Trials J.* **5**, 1015.

REPORT WRITING AND PUBLICATIONS

J. A. Waycott

Doctors who work in the pharmaceutical industry have a particular interest in the publication of original work in scientific journals. This is the principal, and most respectable, means by which essential information about some new compound is circulated. It is on the published evidence that claims are made for the efficacy and safety of a new drug. And it is on these claims that pharmaceutical companies largely base their commercial activities.

In general, of course, the responsibility for the publication of original work lies with the author. But there are occasions, especially for example in the presentation of results from multi-centre trials, when a single individual assumes a co-ordinating role. It is his responsibility to prepare the report in a form suitable for publication. It may also happen that an author needs help in the presentation of his findings. He may not have sufficient time or inclination; his native tongue may not be English. In these circumstances it is natural for him to turn to a colleague better equipped to do the necessary work.

Most of us, at some time or another, have become involved with this process of preparing articles and submitting them for publication. Most of us have approached the matter with some reserve because of its unfamiliarity. We are vaguely aware that there are rules and conventions which, if observed, favour a successful outcome and which, if neglected, may give rise to difficulties. The fact that these so called rules are not at all well remembered makes the whole task rather stressful.

It is my intention now to try and indicate some of the general principles which need to be recognised.

The submission of a paper (other than a review) to a journal normally implies that it presents the results of original research, or some new ideas not previously published; that it is not under consideration for publication elsewhere and that, if accepted, it will not be published anywhere else in the same form, either in English or any other language, without the Editor's consent.

Most editors are very busy. Every article must be gone over in detail; every table and illustration must be examined; precise directions must be given to the printer. Editors have more demands on their available space than they can satisfy. They therefore look favourably on articles presented to them in such a way that no great expenditure of editorial time will be required to put them in order. An article submitted in a careless way, or one that can be made to conform with the usual standards of the journal only with difficulty, may well be set aside. Publication will be delayed or even prevented.

It is important to give a good deal of thought to selecting the most appropriate journal for a particular work. Journals covering a wide range of general interests, and read by workers in all fields of medicine, tend to favour articles that have wide appeal. Journals devoted to narrow interests, on the other hand, are apt to be extremely discriminating in their selection of material.

Having decided on the most suitable journal for the occasion it is prudent (to put it at its lowest) to look within the covers of a back number and see if instructions to intending contributors are available. Many journals issue such instructions. They are not always the same from one journal to the next. Where they are found they should be followed exactly. It is also a necessary precaution to look carefully at the articles that have been published in the journal concerned. The method of presentation should be followed in the draft to be submitted. Some journals, for example, give the summary immediately after the title and authors and before the main text. Others leave the summary to the end and place it immediately before the acknowledgements and references. In some the main headings in the text are placed centrally and in capital letters; in others they are in bold type; and so on. The tables and illustrations should also conform with the pattern favoured by the journals.

The materials to be presented must be clear, precise, logical and brief. A great deal of attention must be given to the way in which the matter is to be set out. Perhaps the most important part of the whole article is the synopsis or summary. This, it must be remembered, is the only part of the paper that will be read by the majority of readers. It must therefore convey with the greatest possible economy and precision the nature of the work described and the most important conclusion or conclusions to emerge.

I shall not refer in detail to the difficulties of writing lucid English with an agreeable style. A nodding acquaintance with the several books written on this subject should be enough to convince anyone that the matter cannot be dealt with properly in a few minutes. If one had to give four rules I think the following would come near the top of the list.

1. Prefer the short to the long word
2. Prefer the Anglo-Saxon to the Romance
3. Use adjectives sparingly
4. Avoid ambiguity and jargon.

It is fashionable in a paper like this to give an example of the kind of writing to avoid and its translation into an acceptable form. The one I have chosen is taken from Bertrand Russell, a man regarded by many as one of the greatest contemporary masters of the English language. Incidentally his maxims for good writing are not exactly the same as those I have just given. He says ' First: never use a long word if a short word will do. Second: if you want to make a statement with a great many qualifications put some of the qualifications in separate sentences. Third: do not let the beginning of your sentence lead the reader to an expectation which is contradicted by the end.'

But to come back to the example of ambiguous and awkward writing. Note the following sentence. 'Human beings are completely exempt from undesirable behaviour-patterns only when certain pre-requisites not satisfied except in a small percentage of actual cases, have, through some fortuitous concourse of favourable circumstances, whether congenital or environmental, chanced to combine in producing an individual in whom many factors deviate from the norm in a socially advantageous manner.' What this means is not immediately obvious. Even when the words are studied carefully their meaning is hard to discover. Russell's attempt to translate this sentence into English reads as follows: 'All men are scoundrels, or at any rate almost all. The men who are not must have had unusual luck, both in their birth and in their upbringing.'

Now in my opinion this is the kind of direct clarity that should be the aim of every writer. His material should be arranged in logical order. There should usually be a short introduction in which the object of the work is stated. The material to be studied and the methods employed should be indicated. Then follows a statement of the results obtained, supported, if necessary, by graphs, histograms, tables or illustrations. The discussion, if any, comes next and the presentation is brought to a close by a concise statement embodying the conclusions to be drawn. I have already mentioned the importance of a properly drafted summary which, conventionally, brings the text of the article to an end. The acknowledgements and the references bring up the rear.

So when it comes to writing a report for publication its outline and probable length should first be settled. Then a rough draft must be prepared. Work on the rough draft eventually reaches the stage at which a preliminary version can be typed. At this stage it is always worthwhile submitting the work to informed criticism by colleagues. In the end a version emerges that is regarded as suitable for submission to the editor of the chosen journal.

For this, clean typescript must be prepared, with double spacing, on sheets of uniform size (generally quarto) and numbered consecutively. The left-hand margin should not be less than 4 cm in width.

The approximate place of tables or illustrations should be marked in the typescript. Tables, figures and illustrations should all be on separate sheets. The legends for these should be collected on another sheet or sheets and identified clearly so that each legend is related to its corresponding figure. Drawings should be prepared in black waterproof ink on a good quality surface. They should be of such a size that after linear reduction to half or a third they will be of the size and shape customary for the journal.

Photographs should be unmounted, glossy, and of high contrast. They should be numbered on the back and marked lightly in pencil with the author's name. The top and bottom of the print should be indicated. Legends should be separate, each clearly related to its proper photograph.

There are two commonly used methods of indicating references in the text of an article. Some journals use one, and some the other, and it is important to set them out in typescript in accordance with the requirements of the journal to which the article is to be submitted. The first method, sometimes called Harvard, gives the names of authors and dates in brackets in the body of the text with the full references arranged alphabetically at the end of the paper. In the second method numbers are used in the text and the references given in numerical order at the end.

Abbreviation of the names of journals should be in accordance with the *World List of Scientific Periodicals* (1963-65), 4th Edition, London, Butterworths.

In conclusion I want to emphasise one or two points that I think are specially important. A good report discloses its meaning with ease and precision. It is written simply and allows no room for pretension of phrase. It is kept as short as possible. In submitting an article for publication the choice of the journal will dictate certain details of presentation. The chances of acceptance are likely to be increased if the article is presented in a form that demands the minimum of editorial time and labour.

THE ROLE OF THE MEDICAL ADVISER IN DRUG EVALUATION

J. D. FITZGERALD

The research departments of pharmaceutical companies function on the hypothesis that new chemical compounds which exhibit activity in a chosen biological system may have a therapeutic application in man.

The medical adviser has the task of determining whether a chemical compound with biological activity has any therapeutic value. This process involves the integration of a number of disciplines with no single discipline being able to carry the work to a final conclusion by itself. The doctor in the Industry plays a central role in this process as an inter-disciplinary coordinator (Fitzgerald, 1968). Not only is he a coordinator but he should also play a creative role (Fig. 1). These roles are best examined separately, though in practice they blend indistinguishably. Undoubtedly the importance of the medical adviser's role varies during the passage of the drug through clinical trial.

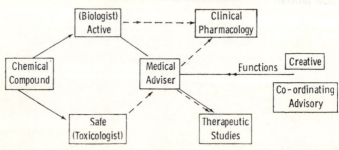

Functions of the Medical Adviser I.

Fig. 1

The inter-relationships of the medical adviser with the phases of drug evaluation.

Creative role

Most large and long established pharmaceutical companies have fairly fixed patterns of research. It is unusual for an individual medical adviser to exert an influence on the general pattern of biological and toxicological research. However, he usually is aware of possible candidate drugs before they are available for study in man. As the compound shows increasing promise he should advise, though this is not always possible, on the details of the toxicological studies. For example in the case of a potential anti-arthritic drug he could emphasise the importance of its effects on the gastro-intestinal tract. Similarly, he should associate closely with the biologist undertaking the animal studies and suggest experiments that may be of significance from a clinical point of view, though not necessarily from other points of view. This early association with the research group can play a decisive part in determining the nature of the contribution the medical adviser makes to the future development of the compound or others in a series. By possessing a secure understanding of the chemistry, pharmacology, pharmacodynamics and toxicology of the drug, the medical adviser can design meaningful studies safely in man and can coordinate and advise with authority.

The initial application of the drug to man is a crucial phase. The object is to determine the presence of biological activity in a new species and to detect unwanted drug-induced effects. The biologist plays an important role at this point and should speak directly to the investigator carrying out the human studies. The medical adviser plays a subsidiary role in the phase of external pharmacology. The investigator chosen for the study is normally an expert in the particular field. The collaboration is ideally between experts in different species. However, the investigator may be one of two kinds: (1) a disease expert and (2) a pharmacodynamic expert.

In the first instance, the medical adviser may need to supply expertise on, for example, the type of screening for organ toxicity, the timing and treatment of blood and urine samples for assay of the new drug. If the investigator is more pharmacodynamically orientated, the medical adviser can suggest the type of patient material that will give the greatest amount of meaningful information in the quickest time and with the least number of subjects. In either event, the medical adviser must constantly keep ethical considerations in mind in relation to the experimental protocols designed by the biologist and clinical investigator.

At this early phase, the medical adviser can add considerably to the understanding of the new compound by carrying out his own pharmacodynamic studies in the human. Some recent work with a new adrenergic beta receptor blocking drug provides a useful example (Fitzgerald and Scales, 1968). Preliminary studies in man had shown that this drug was active parenterally in angina pectoris and cardiac arrhythmias. Whilst awaiting permission to arrange chronic oral studies in these indications, a study in healthy volunteers was carried out to determine (1) the half-life of the drug given orally, (2) the nature of the urinary metabolites, (3) the blood level that would inhibit an exercise tachycardia and (4) the daily oral dose necessary to achieve this blood level. Tests were also carried out for evidence of organ toxicity. Thus when permission was received to extend clinical trials in patients much time and unnecessary work in patients was saved by knowledge of the dose, blood levels and metabolites. The medical adviser is in a unique position to perform such studies since only he will have available the requisite knowledge, expertise and equipment at that point in time.

Once the phase of demonstrating a degree of safety and activity is passed, further progress is determined to a considerable degree by the competence and application of the medical adviser, It is clear from the preceding chapters how much creative and objective thought goes into the design of a clinical trial. The medical adviser is the person who decides *what* questions need to be answered about the drug, the *order* in which the answers needs to be obtained and, in consultation with his investigators, *the manner* in which the questions are answered. Thus these days the medical adviser to an extent selects or rejects proposed studies. It is at this phase that the adviser should be most creative. To take a simple example, in the case of a beta blocking agent, he decides whether initial investigations are carried out in angina pectoris or in phaeochromocytoma. He decides whether the initial studies answer the question, does this beta blocker increase exercise tolerance or should answer the question, does this drug relieve anginal pain? These decisions will determine which investigator is first approached and how the studies are designed.

Coordinating and advisory function

Once a drug shows therapeutic promise more trials commence in many centres both at home and abroad. It is no longer possible for the medical adviser to maintain the intimate contact that is achieved with the initial investigators. At this phase his role evolves into one of coordination and advice (Fig. 2). It is unfortunate that some clinicians still believe that the function of the medical adviser is merely to ensure that adequate supplies of clinical material arrive at the right place at the right time.

Functions of the Medical Adviser II.

Creative.	Co-ordinating and Advisory.
Internal Clinical Pharmacology.	Selection of investigators.
	Statistical advice.
Clinical trial design.	Trial execution.
	eg. Dose schedule.
	Drug coding.
	Formulation.
	Record sheets.
	Compilation of results.
	Monitoring side effects.
	Ethical aspects.
	Drug authority documentation.
	Marketing advice.

FIG. 2

Summary of the creative and advisory functions
of the medical adviser.

The medical adviser should be the person who poses the outstanding questions that need answering. He should also give guidance on the statistical aspects governing the trial's design and also advise investigators *not* to do a trial because it is statistically invalid. Furthermore, alterations in the formulation, dose and route of administration of a drug are sometimes required. No one else is really in a position to advise with authority on these matters. Many of the investigators involved in this phase of the study are primarily clinicians who are disease orientated rather than drug orientated.

Hence the medical adviser is relied upon to provide guidance on the direction of trials and also on the ethical aspects of the studies. For example, he may be contacted by an investigator who is not equipped to undertake clinical trials. The role of the adviser in this situation is to prevent trials taking place which are not likely to give valid information. He also is increasingly concerned with monitoring the feed back of data on the screening tests for organ toxicity. In addition, he serves as the first relay station for obtaining data on unwanted side effects communicating it to other investigators working with the drug and informing the health authorities as required.

The degree to which the medical adviser succeeds in this difficult role of coordinator and adviser depends on a number of factors. Firstly, it should be clear to his investigators that he is fully competent in the field in which the studies are to be carried out. It is essential that a degree of mutual respect is achieved between the medical adviser and the investigator. This is most easily developed by demonstrating a complete understanding of the drug and intellectual honesty. The medical adviser should indicate that his attitude to his work is to assist in the discovery of therapeutic agents, to ensure that they are correctly used and that his company derives the maximum benefit in the most ethical fashion.

The final aim of the work is to obtain a drug that can be marketed. To assist in this, the medical adviser is in a position to offer the investigator financial assistance if required in order to carry the work through. The time should be long passed when the object of such financial grants is misconstrued.

The performance of a clinical trial not only involves the pharmaceutical company in financial expenditure, but will frequently involve the investigator in expense.

The most modest financial outlay occurs, for example, in the cost of printing record forms and arranging for special labelling of containers. Again, special apparatus may need to be purchased to enable the trialist to carry out the less common types of investigation. These expenses should be borne by the pharmaceutical company concerned.

Many doctors or their technical assistants have to devote much additional time to ensure the adequate progress of a trial. In such circumstances, the persons involved should receive payment for the additional service they provide. It is essential that the clinical trials doctor makes it clear that whatever financial cost is incurred by the trial will be paid whatever the outcome of the study. There is no doubt that misunderstandings do occasionally arise on both sides over this aspect of clinical trials. This should not occur if the medical adviser clarifies his attitude to financial grants to assist investigators at an early stage in the initiation of a trial. Finally, the medical adviser provides valuable help in writing reports or preparing papers relating to the clinical studies. The degree to which he participates in the preparation of papers varies from suggesting the skeleton of the paper to preparing a final draft for consideration by the authors. A careful analysis and compilation of all trials data must be made by the medical adviser. His final opinion will strongly influence any marketing decisions. He must prepare, therefore, a ' Platform ' or guide describing the drug's merits, side effects, precautions and contraindications. The practising doctor relies on this advice and opinion when prescribing the drug. Similarly, the Platform guides sales managers, trainers and representatives, as to what can and cannot be said about the drug. This is one of the most responsible and least recognised aspects of a medical adviser's role. In future his advice may well carry legal responsibility in Great Britain under the provision of the Medicines Act (1968).

An experienced medical adviser is an invaluable asset to the medical profession as well as to the pharmaceutical industry. He provides the vital link between basic organised research and the field of clinical medicine. He must be competent as a clinician and have an above average understanding of pharmacology, pharmacodynamics, statistics and toxicology.

He must ensure that his work conforms to the highest standards of ethical practice. The importance of his role is summarised in Figure 3. In regard to personal qualities, he should be intelligent, honest and have a well rounded personality which enables him to work with many sorts of persons and enables differing personalities to collaborate with each other to achieve a common aim.

Many persons may feel that they have never met this idealised medical adviser. Thus the wider issue arises as to how doctors can be trained to be competent medical advisers. Before entering the Pharmaceutical industry, formal training in clinical pharmacology is desirable but not essential. However, three to five years hospital training is desirable.

As with most specialities in medicine, practical experience is the best way to become competent.

I would suggest that the medical adviser should be trained within the Industry. The following scheme summarises my personal view of the form of training (Fig. 4).

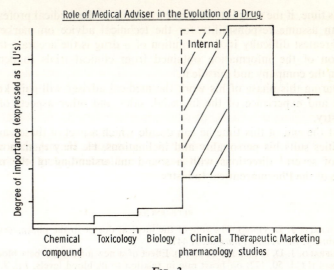

FIG. 3

The varying importance of the medical adviser's role in the
evolution of a drug.

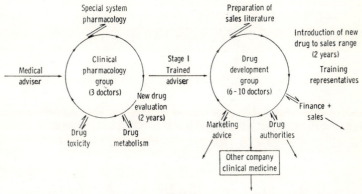

FIG. 4

Proposed scheme for the training of medical advisers. The unidirectional
arrows indicate the future responsibilities at the end of the period of
training.

The time scale is three to five years. On entering the industry the
new adviser should be attached to a clinical pharmacology group
comprising two or three doctors experienced in drug evaluation.
During this period of one or two years the adviser may assist an
experienced doctor in evaluating a new drug. He should be given the
opportunity to acquire an understanding of the principles of drug
toxicity, drug metabolism and stage I drug evaluation. At the end

of this time, if the drug is to be made available to the medical profession he can assume responsibility for the technical advice on marketing. The greatest difficulty in the evolution of a drug is the accurate transmission of the information obtained from clinical trials to persons within the company and outside it.

During this phase of his work the medical adviser will gain knowledge and experience of the financial, sales and other aspects of the Industry.

At the end of this time he can decide which aspect of these various activities suits his personality and inclinations. He may then move in one of several directions with a sound understanding of the many facets of the Pharmaceutical Industry.

REFERENCES

FITZGERALD, J. D. (1968). The role of the medical doctor in the pharmaceutical industry. *Int. J. clin. Pharmac.* **1,** 447.

FITZGERALD, J. D. & SCALES, B. (1968). Effect of a new adrenergic beta blocking agent (I.C.I. 50, 172) on heart rate in relation to its blood levels. *Int. J. clin. Pharmac.* **1,** 467.

Part II

PRACTICAL APPLICATION

CARDIOVASCULAR DRUG EVALUATION

(1) HYPERTENSION

W. I. CRANSTON

Previous papers have dealt with theoretical aspects of clinical trials, and with the practical problems common to all kinds of controlled trials. I shall limit myself to trials in the field of hypertension, with particular reference to the comparison of different drugs.

There is good evidence that treatment of hypertension improves the outlook in patients with diastolic blood pressures in excess of 120 mm Hg (Leishman, 1963; Hamilton *et al.*, 1964; Veteran's Administration, 1967). Previous cardiac or cerebrovascular disease does not contraindicate treatment.

Measurement of blood pressure

Technical aspects. There are several technical problems in the measurement of blood pressure. An extensive discussion of these problems is given by Rose *et al.* (1964). Many of them can be overcome by the use of sphygmomanometers in which the observer makes a decision about the level of arterial pressure without knowing at the time the absolute pressure level. There are two types of machines of this kind. On the first, the observer arrests the fall of mercury in a column, at the time when he hears the appearance of sounds. In parallel mercury columns, he arrests the fall of the mercury when he hears muffling and disappearance of sounds. Only after the completion of this operation does he read off the systolic and diastolic blood pressures (Rose *et al.*, 1964). This type of machine avoids many of the errors inherent in ordinary blood pressure measurements but it is rather cumbersome, and weighs over 25 lb. The other type of machine is less clumsy, though slightly more open to some errors. With this machine the observer measures blood pressure in the ordinary way; at the end of the operation the mercury does not return to zero, and the final mercury level must be subtracted from the measured values to give the true blood pressure reading. The zero shift is changed between observations, and the observer has no foreknowledge of the magnitude of the zero shift (Garrow, 1963). There is no doubt that clinical trials of any hypotensive agent should always be carried out using apparatus which avoids observer bias.

At the beginning of every trial, if more than one observer is taking part, it must be clearly agreed whether phase IV or phase V of the Korotoff sounds will be used to determine diastolic pressure. Which is used is not too important; though phase IV may give a slightly better estimate of true diastolic pressure, phase V may be easier to measure. A further small technical point concerns the design of blood pressure cuff, and the influence of arm circumference on blood pressure levels by sphygmomanometry. There has been some disagreement over the years about the influence of arm circumference on the accuracy of blood pressure measurement using sphygmomanometry.

The influence of width of the cuff on this error has been widely examined, but not the influence of cuff length, though this was mentioned in 1905 (Martin, 1905). Recently King (1967) has shown that a great deal of the cuff artifact is due to failure of the balloon within the cuff to encircle the arm completely. There is a strong case for using a bladder 42 cm long, rather than the standard length of 22 or 26 cm, in all sphygmomanometers, and certainly in those employed in clinical trials.

Physiological aspects. Turning now to more physiological variables one of the main problems is the variability of blood pressure. Which blood pressure should one take and when? Figure 1 shows the spontaneous variation in arterial pressure over several hours in a patient with fairly severe essential hypertension. Apart from the marked fall with sleep, there is a considerable variation from time to time during

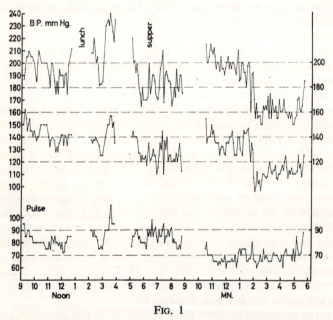

FIG. 1

Diurnal variation in arterial blood pressure measured automatically in a patient with hypertension. (Reproduced with permission from Richardson, D. W., Honour, A. J., Fenton, G. W., Stott, F. H. and Pickering, G. W. (1964) *Clin. Sci.* **26,** 445.)

the day. It is not yet practical to get numerous, repeated or continuous blood pressure measurements from patients living a normal life. Though in theory this might be ideal, it would involve quite complex problems of data handling. Thus one must compromise, and measure the patient's blood pressure as often as one can, but in circumstances that are as unchanging as possible. The repeated recording of arterial pressure may have its own effects, however, as is shown in Figure 2. This patient had her blood pressure recorded at weekly intervals while receiving placebo tablets. Her arterial pressure fell from 210/120 mm Hg to 155/90. This, of course, would have been a splendid therapeutic effect if any supposedly active agent had been given. In this patient, who shows the phenomenon to an unusual extent, the maximum change occurred around 6 weeks. There is clearly a strong case for a 'run in' period in any field of the less potent hypertensive drugs, using placebos, in order to detect this kind of patient. It is impossible to say how long it should be, and here again compromise is called for. We have usually allowed a 3-week run-in period, and have thereafter checked blood pressure changes for trend with time, independent of the nature of the treatment given.

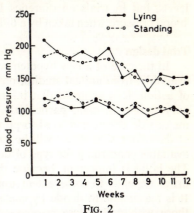

FIG. 2

Arterial pressure measured at weekly intervals on an outpatient receiving inert tablets. (Reproduced with permission from Pickering, G. W., Cranston, W. I. and Pears, M. A. (1961) *The Treatment of Hypertension*. Charles C. Thomas, Springfield, Illinois.)

The time of day when the patient is seen is of great importance if one is assessing drugs which interfere with autonomic transmission. There is evidence that hypertensive patients show an exaggerated diurnal swing in blood volume (Cranston and Brown, 1962); in the afternoon their plasma volume is about 10 per cent higher than in the morning. Patients with sympathetic blockade are extremely sensitive to small changes of blood volume, so that afternoon blood pressure usually tends to be higher than morning blood pressure. Thus, in any trial in which dosage is titrated to induce a given blood pressure reduction, it will be easier to attain the objective in the morning than in the afternoon. Clearly, if the same patient is seen at different times on different occasions, the precision of any average value is going to decrease, and indeed misleading results may be obtained. The other variable is the observer. Ideally, all blood pressures on any patient should be taken by the same observer. This is a policy of perfection and again, some times compromise is necessary. In one trial on autonomic blocking agents (Prichard *et al.*, 1968), it was found that substitution of an observer did not significantly affect blood pressure levels, but in trials on diuretics I have seen quite large increases in blood pressure when taken by a different observer.

Trial design

In the case of a new hypotensive drug, adequate evidence should be available, from animal studies, on its effectiveness and probable mode of action. It is assumed that information is also available on preliminary studies in man, particularly on the drug's dose response curve, major side effects and its absorption and excretion. By this stage, some of the major side effects will be known, and some information will be available concerning the type of dose response curve of blood pressure. The latter is important, because the critical assessment of hypotensive drugs depends to some extent upon the way in which the drug acts. It is reasonable to divide hypotensive agents into two general types—those with a flat dose response curve, and those with a steep dose response curve. Examples of the former include diuretics and Rauwolfia compounds, and of the latter, all of the autonomic blocking agents. For purposes of brevity I shall arbitrarily term these non-titratable and titratable agents. Non-titratable drugs do not usually require meticulous attention to dosage and their effects, in general, are manifest rather slowly—over a period of days or weeks rather than hours. Their effects on arterial pressure are generally less dramatic than those of the titratable drugs.

Titratable drugs. Controlled clinical trials of titratable drugs are more difficult to carry out than trials of non-titratable drugs, because the dose has to be determined and regulated for each patient. With this kind of drug, there is a strong case for assessing the agent initially in an uncontrolled way, in a limited number of centres. This will give some experience of how to use the drug, the incidence of severe side effects, the range of dosage required, and the likelihood of any form of toxicity not revealed in the initial pilot study. Some potentially toxic actions may still remain concealed, as for example the development of a lupus erythematosus syndrome with hydralazine (Morrow *et al.*, 1953), or the appearance of positive Coomb's tests with methyldopa (Carstairs *et al.*, 1966).

With titratable drugs it will usually be possible to effect a large reduction, at least for some time, in the level of blood pressure of most hypertensive patients, and in a controlled trial the object will be to achieve a predetermined blood pressure level for each patient. In all controlled trials of hypotensive drugs the patient should act as his own control and should receive, in random sequence, all of the drugs under examination. This means that variation between patients is eliminated. This type of trial will usually be conducted upon patients with fairly severe hypertension because it is this type of patient who will usually be treated with the titratable type of drug. As in any trial, the criteria for selection of patients must be clearly defined. Important points include the age, sex, blood pressure levels untreated, renal function, and evidence of vascular disease. Patients with hypertension secondary to treatable disease should usually be excluded, but those with bilateral renal disease, for example, may be included. They may need to be treated as a separate group, but this is usually unnecessary. One particularly important aspect of patient selection is some assessment of their likely co-operation. In comparative trials of this sort patients should be told exactly what the problems are and how the trial is to be run. Most trials will require frequent attendances by the patients, over a period of several months at least, and it is important not only to obtain the patient's cooperation but to assess how reliable he will be. One way of doing this is to test the patient's reliability in a pre-trial period, as was done in the Veterans' Administration combined trial on the effects of treatment on morbidity and hypertension (1967). This has the disadvantage of lengthening the whole trial period and this must be weighed against the advantages. With this kind of trial, no placebo period should be employed, because the withdrawal of treatment may be dangerous in patients with severe hypertension. The agents under examination must be compared with agents whose effectiveness is known. Each drug must be titrated in an attempt to reach a predetermined blood pressure level, which need not be the same for all patients. For example, it may be decided that a diastolic pressure of 100 mm Hg may be the objective for patients aged over 55, and 90 mm Hg for patients under this age. The objectives may be quite flexible, to allow for the views of the physicians concerned in the trial. The important point is that they should be agreed and clearly set out before the trial begins. It should also be remembered that the more complex the design, the greater the risk of errors. Particularly with agents which interfere with autonomic transmission, it must be decided whether the desired blood pressure should be measured with the patient standing or recumbent. There is at present no valid evidence, in therapeutic terms, to show whether it is essential to reduce recumbent blood pressure to any fixed level, and in practice there is a good deal to be said for aiming at a given blood pressure level with the patient standing up. Both types of approach have been used (Vejlsgaard *et al.*, 1967; Prichard *et al.*, 1968). In considering any drug for treatment of hypertension, the object is to reduce blood pressure without causing side effects. In comparing titratable drugs the desired blood pressure level is set, and the 'measured variables' are the number of patients in whom control cannot be achieved, whether because of ineffectiveness or because of side effects, and the relative severity of side effects in patients achieving the desired level of control. There are good arguments for operating a trial of this kind with two independent observers, in order that bias may be eliminated without danger of overdosage. In principle an observer, ignorant of the drug the patient is receiving, should measure the blood pressure and determine whether the patient's future dosage should be increased, decreased or unaltered. The second observer should enquire about side effects (since the nature of the side effects may give some clue to the treatment being employed), and may decide the size of increment of dose. There is growing evidence that written questionnaires may be at least as accurate, and perhaps more accurate, than questioning for side effects, but this has not been conclusively determined. A written questionnaire will not easily distinguish spontaneous complaints from those elicited by questioning, but it does eliminate any unconscious bias on the part of the observer. Whether the second observer should also be ignorant of the drugs used is a moot point. Particularly if one drug has distinctive side effects, it may be impossible for him to be ' blind ' and Prichard *et al.* (1968) advance arguments for the second observer being aware of the treatment used. Nevertheless, Vejlsgaard *et al.* (1967) did conduct a trial of this type with the second observer ignorant of the treatment used. The most important comparison between drugs is in the severity of unwanted effects; with the exception of weight changes, postural and exercise hypotension and evidence, if any, of biological or haematological changes, unwanted effects are all subjective and there is no entirely satisfactory way of handling this information. In a general sense the more side effects, the worse the drug, and if there is a very clearcut difference between drugs, the answer may be self-evident. In some trials different side effects have been allocated scores; it is arguable that this may, in fact, confuse the issue because it introduces an arbitrary index of relative severity. In this type of trial there is an initial period of variable duration with each drug, while the dose of the drug is increased until the desired blood pressure level is reached, or until it is clear that the desired blood pressure level cannot be attained with the drug in question. Thereafter the patient is treated with each agent for an arbitrary period of time to ensure that control can be maintained. The time period has usually been 2 to 3 months in trials of this type. Clearly, if patients require to have their hypertension treated, they require to have their blood pressures controlled indefinitely, and a theoretical argument can be made for continuing these trials for a very long time. Practical difficulties militate against this, as does the consideration that the natural history of the illness may change; there is evidence that some patients who have had severe hypertension treated for years, may sustain a low level of blood pressure when treatment is withdrawn.

Another variable which may be included in trials of titratable drugs is non-titratable drugs. Here again, the decision whether to use those agents is in the hands of the investigator. In Vejlsgaard's trial (1967), all patients remained on a fixed dose of diuretics throughout the study. In the trial reported by Prichard *et al.* (1968) diuretics were added to the regimen, for each primary drug, if it was impossible to maintain blood pressure control with the primary drug alone.

In the last four years, three comparative trials of titratable sympathetic blocking agents have been carried out. One was not controlled (Oates *et al.*, 1965) and two were (Vejlsgaard *et al.*, 1967; Pritchard *et al.*, 1968). Though different drugs were used, guanethidine and methyldopa were included on all three comparisons. When one considers the difficulties involved in trials of this kind, the concordance of view about the relative merits of methyldopa and guanethidine is both surprising and reassuring.

Non-titratable drugs. These agents, as already mentioned, have flat dose-response curves and are relatively less potent than titratable drugs. It is therefore not possible to aim at a certain blood pressure level and to assess the difficulty of achieving it.

They are generally less potent than titratable drugs and, because their effect usually takes some time to be manifest, they should be subject to controlled trials relatively early in their careers. Since the response curve is flat, it is much simpler to design trials for these drugs, using one or more fixed levels of dosage. Here the dependent variable is the change of blood pressure, and the evidence of side effects. This type of trial can best be done in patients with less severe hypertension. Once again, each patient should act as his own control. With this kind of drug, it is important to include at least one placebo period, and perhaps more, in the assessment period; if the drug under trial has less hypotensive action than an established agent, it is impossible to tell whether it is completely ineffective unless a placebo period is included. The inclusion of a placebo period will also provide evidence about the validity of complaints of side effects.

In our hands the results of this kind of trial have been remarkably reproducible (Cranston *et al.*, 1963; Cranston *et al.*, 1965). When the same dose of the same drug has been used in different trials very similar results have been obtained. The same kind of trial design can be employed, when assessing the additive effect of non-titratable drugs in the presence of established doses of titratable drugs (Juel-Jenson and Pears, 1960).

The imponderables in this type of trial are similar to those in trials of titratable drugs. There is, for example, no simple answer to the duration of each treatment block, and the comparison of side effects may be difficult.

Problems

Discrepancies. Though one can arbitrarily divide drugs into titratable and non-titratable groups, it is important to ensure that any drug has the right kind of trial. There is reasonable agreement between the results of trials on titratable agents, as previously mentioned, and also between different trials of non-titratable agents.

11

One agent, whose efficacy remains a matter of controversy, is propranolol. This drug has been examined in several trials of the non-titratable type, and in these circumstances has been generally found unimpressive (Paterson and Dollery, 1966; Richardson *et al.*, 1968). The main reports of its effectiveness have come from those using the drug in a titratable fashion (Prichard and Gillam, 1969). No properly controlled trial has been carried out with propranolol used in this way, and it is possible that some of the discrepancies arise from subjecting the drug to the wrong kind of trial.

Tablet taking. It is clearly important to know whether patients are actually taking tablets prescribed. All sorts of methods have been proposed for determining this, but none is entirely satisfactory.

If one is reasonably assured of the patient's cooperation, merely asking the patient about his tablet consumption has advantages. If the patient is going to 'cheat' he will probably be able to circumvent any scheme to test his co-operation. The methods that have been employed include tablet counts, and the incorporation of riboflavin (5 mg) into placebo tablets (Veterans Administration, 1967). It is also important to control, or at least to be aware of, the patient's consumption of other drugs. For example, tricyclic antidepressants can interfere markedly with the hypotensive action of many sympathetic efferent blocking agents (Mitchell *et al.*, 1967).

References

CARSTAIRS, K. C., BRECKENRIDGE, A., DOLLERY, C. T. & WORLLEDGE, S. M. (1966). Incidence of a positive direct Coomb's test in patients on α-methyldopa. *Lancet,* **2,** 133.

CRANSTON, W. I. & BROWN, W. (1962). Diurnal variation in plasma volume in normal and hypertensive subjects. *Clin. Sci.* **25,** 107.

CRANSTON, W. I., JUEL-JENSEN, B. E., SEMMENCE, A. M., HANDFIELD-JONES, R. P. C., FORBES, J. A. & MUTCH, L. M. M. (1963). Effects of oral diuretics on raised arterial pressure. *Lancet,* **2,** 966.

CRANSTON, W. I., SEMMENCE, A. M., RICHARDSON, D. W. & BARNETT, C. F. (1965). Effect of triamterene on elevated arterial pressure. *Am. Heart J.* **70,** 455.

GARROW, J. S. (1963). Zero-muddler for unprejudiced sphygmomanometry. *Lancet,* **2,** 1205.

HAMILTON, M., THOMPSON, E. N. & WISNIEWSKI, T. K. M. (1964). Role of blood pressure control in preventing complications of hypertension. *Lancet,* **1,** 235.

JUEL-JENSEN, B. E. & PEARS, M. A. (1960). Chlorothiazide in treatment of high blood-pressure. Results of a controlled trial. *Br. med J.* **1,** 523.

KING, G. E. (1967). Errors in clinical measurement of blood pressure in obesity. *Clin. Sci.* **32,** 223.

LEISHMAN, A. W. D. (1963). Merits of reducing high blood pressure. *Lancet,* **1,** 1284.

MARTIN, C. J. (1905). The determination of arterial blood pressure in clinical practice. *Br. med. J.* **1,** 865.

MITCHELL, J. R., ARIAS, L. & OATES, J. A. (1967). Antagonism of the antihypertensive action of guanethidine sulphate by desipramine hydrochloride. *J. Am. med. Ass.* **202,** 973.

MORROW, J. D., SCHROEDER, H. A. & PERRY, H. M. (1953). Studies on the control of hypertension by Hyphex. *Circulation,* **8,** 829.

OATES, J. A., SELIGMANN, A. W., CLARK, M. A., ROUSSIAN, P. & LEE, R. E. (1965). The relative efficacy of guanethidine, methyldopa and pargyline as antihypertensive agents. *New Engl. J. Med.,* **273,** 729.

PATERSON, J. W. & DOLLERY, C. T. (1966). Effect of propranolol in mild hypertension. *Lancet,* **2,** 1148.

PRICHARD, B. N. C. & GILLAM, P. M. S. (1969). Treatment of hypertension with propranolol. *Br. med. J.* **1,** 7.

PRICHARD, B. N. C., JOHNSON, A. W., HILL, I. D. & ROSENHEIM, M. (1968). Bethanidine, guanethidine and methyldopa in treatment of hypertension: a within patient comparison. *Br. med. J.* **1,** 135.

RICHARDSON, D. W., FRIEND, J., GEAR, A. S., MAUCK, H. P. & PRESTON, L. W. (1968). Effect of propranolol on elevated arterial pressure. *Circulation,* **37,** 534.

ROSE, G. A., HOLLAND, W. W. & CROWLEY, E. A. (1964). A sphygmomanometer for epidemiologists. *Lancet,* **1,** 296.

VEJLSGAARD, V., CHRISTENSEN, M. & CLAUSEN, E. (1967). Double blind trial of four hypotensive drugs (methyldopa and three sympatholytic agents). *Br. med. J.* **2,** 598.

VETERANS' ADMINISTRATION CO-OPERATIVE STUDY GROUP ON ANTIHYPERTENSIVE AGENTS (1967). Effects of treatment of morbidity in hypertension. *J. Am. med. Ass.* **202,** 1028.

CARDIOVASCULAR DRUG EVALUATION

(2) THE ASSESSMENT OF ANTI-ANGINAL DRUGS

G. E. SOWTON and J. D. FITZGERALD

Introduction

A reliable assessment of the clinical value and mode of action of a new drug for the treatment of angina pectoris is of immense importance to the patient, to the practising physician and to the pharmaceutical manufacturer, yet a review of the world literature will show that this is rarely achieved. In this paper we discuss some of the problems which beset the assessement of such drugs and suggest the lines on which trials of new compounds might be organised.

We shall consider only those drugs which are intended to treat or prevent attacks of angina pectoris provoked by any of the usual stimuli on patients with coronary heart disease. We exclude drugs intended to influence the underlying pathological condition of the heart, or to treat patients whose angina is due to other causes such as syphilitic ostial stenosis, aortic stenosis, cardiomyopathy or ventricular tachycardia. We emphasise that the term ' anti-anginal drug ' is not the same as ' coronary vasodilator '. There is considerable evidence that coronary vasodilation contributes little to the relief of anginal chest pain.

AIMS OF AN ANTI-ANGINAL TRIAL

Assessment of a new drug should provide answers to the following questions: (1) Is it effective? (2) Is it safe? (3) How does it act? (4) How does it compare with established drugs? These questions can be answered by evaluation of the drugs in three stages.

Stage 1. Preliminary trials with intravenous administration in a small number of patients.

Stage 2. Controlled trials with oral administration of both drugs and placebo to a moderate number of patients.

Stage 3. Large scale trials in many centres over a prolonged period.

STAGES OF EVALUATION

Stage 1

This concerns the testing of a new drug in man for the first time. The object of these studies is to determine the effect of acute short-term administration on resting and exercise haemodynamics and on effort tolerance. They are intended to provide an indication that the drug has no untoward haemodynamic effects in man, that when given in the correct dose it increases exercise tolerance and possibly improves the ECG during effort and to establish the broad range of doses within which therapeutic effects may be expected.

At this stage a single blind technique is satisfactory, the drug being given intravenously and compared with normal saline. Only a small number of patients need be included, but they should have typical angina which has been stable for several months and which should be due to coronary heart disease without complicating factors such as recent myocardial infarction, dysrhythmias, valve disease or heart failure. The procedure including the exercise tests must be carefully explained to such patients and informed consent obtained.

A standard exercise test is the most satisfactory means of assessing drugs at this stage and most information is obtained from a test in which the patient exercises until stopped by pain. The exercise can be carried out on a treadmill, a bicycle ergometer or by a standard procedure such as the two-step test. It must be recognised that every exercise test in a patient with angina involves some risk but it appears justifiable to exercise the patient until ECG signs of ischaemia or the presence of chest pain limits exercise, since the onset of pain is the symptom which brought the patient to the doctor. In fact an exercise test of similar severity is carried out by the patient during his everyday life whenever he experiences anginal pain. There is, however, a major difference in the circumstances of the anginal pain between outside and inside hospital. In hospital, the test is performed under controlled conditions with an ECG available and an experienced physician with resuscitation equipment to hand in the event of any dysrhythmia.

It is important that whichever exercise test is chosen the subject is familiar with the type of exercise and a trial run is advisable. In case of exercise on a treadmill or ergometer in particular, a warm-up period is recommended since the results may otherwise be invalid. It has been shown in relatively normal subjects that haemodynamic measurements and indices of cardiac work (such as the tension time index and LV external work) are not reproducible during the second of two identical exercise periods separated by one hour of rest (Burkart et al., 1967). If a patient is therefore exercised as a control run, given a drug and then re-exercised a false impression of the activity of the drug may be obtained. In most instances the LV work is lower at a comparable exercise level during the second exercise period and this results in an apparent increase in exercise tolerance due to the drug under test (Fig. 1).

There is no reason to suppose that these results do not also apply to patients with angina and coronary heart disease, and so the use of saline injections in at least some of the exercise tests is essential if an accurate conclusion is to be reached. The differences are considerably less between the second and third periods of exercise than between the first and second, so that the inclusion of a preliminary warm-up period reduces error from this cause.

For the initial few patients it is preferable for the haemodynamic effects of the drug to be assessed without the exercise level being

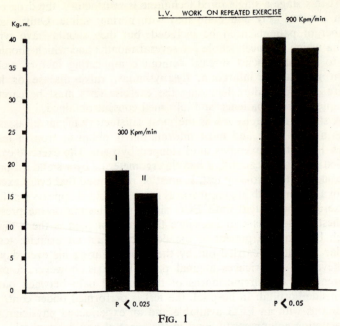

FIG. 1

The calculated LV work was higher during the first of two identical periods of exercise on a bicycle ergometer both at 300 kpm/min. and at 900 kpm/min. The exercise periods were separated by one hour.

sufficient to produce anginal pain. A suitable trial design is for two injections of the drug to be given during ' steady state ' exercise at a level of about 300 kpm/min. (equivalent to running slowly) on a bicycle ergometer. The changes after the first injection are compared with those after the second. Even a third injection may be incorporated so that a primitive type of dose-response curve is obtained (Gibson et al., 1970). During the next series of patients in Stage 1 of the investigation the exercise level should be such that pain is produced fairly soon after the start of exercise. The maximal cardiac load is usually achieved within two to three minutes after the beginning of exercise and subsequent haemodynamic changes tend to reduce cardiac work for a constant exercise level (Sowton and Burkart, 1967). Alterations in the rate of change of these variables may mask minor drug effects and incorrect conclusions be reached about the activity of the drug under test. It is possible to design a trial so that the effects of double exercise changes are eliminated by a series of repeat exercise tests with random dosing of saline controls and the drug under test (Conway et al., 1968). This involves several attendances for each patient and many dozen exercise tests before valid conclusions can be reached. It is doubtful if this procedure is justified in Stage 1 trials.

Ideally, the test should be carried out at a fixed time after the last meal and at a constant room temperature which should be the same from day to day. Patients should not smoke on the day of the test and the test should be postponed if trinitrin has been taken during the last four hours.

An ideal approach would also involve training the patient with repeated exercise tests daily for 8 to 10 days until exercise tolerance is constant and the patient is well used to the test machine. The definitive investigation can then be carried out following the standard warm-up procedure. This is extremely expensive in terms of time for the patient, the laboratory and the investigator and is probably unnecessary for a Stage 1 investigation. The method is valuable for definitive investigation of the haemodynamic effects of drugs (Chamberlain, 1966).

Stage 1 trials of this type should be accompanied by determination of the blood levels of the drug so that the haemodynamic and clinical effects can be related to the rate of absorption, and the half life, as well as the clinical response to different blood concentrations. The findings can then be assessed as a whole to determine the blood levels to be achieved by oral medication if the drug is taken on to Stage 2 trials.

Stage 2

This will only be carried out if the drug has been shown to be effective and safe during Stage 1 studies and when the oral doses necessary to achieve satisfactory blood levels have been determined.

The object of Stage 2 studies is to determine the effect of long term oral administration of the drug on the incidence of anginal pain. The studies are also designed to assess the side effects and toxicity associated with oral administration in man.

Selection of patients. As before patients should have angina pectoris due to coronary heart disease and should be in a ' stable phase ', i.e. the severity of the pain should not have altered significantly during the last four months. Patients should have at least one typical attack of anginal pain each day, should be good observers and should be able to describe accurately the character and severity of the pain. They should be able to appreciate the development of side effects and any change in their daily exercise tolerance produced by the drug. As before they should appreciate that they are participating in an investigation and informed consent must be obtained.

Trial design. It is now generally agreed that the double blind cross over study should be used for Stage 2 trials (Batterman and Grossman, 1955). There is less agreement as to the dosage schedule indicated. If the trial can be designed so that each patient receives the drug at three different dose levels chosen to cover the expected therapeutic range, then it is likely that a satisfactory result will be achieved. Alternatively the individual dose for each patient may be determined during a preliminary period and the trial proper started only when this has been found. This second scheme assumes that the drug is active since the physician only accepts that an adequate dose has been reached when the patient is relieved of symptoms and it is therefore probably better to include a range of doses for every patient. Nevertheless, it is important that each patient enters the trial with a 'run-in' period in order that the placebo effects and the well-known reduction in anginal pain at the onset of every trial may be avoided (Evans and Hoyle, 1933; Beecher, 1955; Cole and Griffiths, 1958). Ideally, this 'run-in' period should be as long as possible—three months is recommended—but in practice this may unduly prolong the trial and make it administratively inconvenient, so that a one month 'run-in' period is usually acceptable.

A suitable trial design is for each patient to receive treatment packs covering 2 to 4 weeks' supply of active drug and placebo distributed on a randomised basis. At each attendance he is then asked to express his preference in terms of reduction of anginal attacks and perhaps also in terms of well-being, increase in effort tolerance, or other criteria of effect (such as frequency of attacks noted in a diary, or trinitrin tablets remaining) at his next attendance. This procedure is repeated using treatment packs containing higher doses of drug until the patient has received three complete periods of treatment and has been reviewed at the end of each period. A full history, clinical examination, 12 lead ECG and exercise test should be carried out on each attendance and the results evaluated in parallel but independently from the subjective preference of the patient.

Assessment. Trials involving small numbers of patients should be avoided since a highly biased result in either direction may be obtained. The results are evaluated statistically either when the trial is completed by all patients or on sequential basis in which preferences are plotted on a chart as each patient completes the trial (Armitage, 1954). In either case it is unlikely that a clear cut answer will be achieved by a trial involving less than 20 or 30 patients and each measurement chosen as criterion of efficacy (i.e. patient's preference, exercise tolerance, ECG improvement) must be evaluated separately. Statistical significance at the 5 per cent level is satisfactory and the temptation to report 'trends' which do not achieve this level of significance must be resisted. Side-effects and pathological changes (such as alterations in the white cell count) are listed and analysed separately according to whether they arose during active or placebo therapy.

Multiple centre trials. It is advisable that such Stage 2 studies should be carried out by several investigators in different centres throughout the country and possibly in different countries. By taking a large number of patients in this way a broader spectrum of the effects of the drug will be achieved. In particular it is likely that the development of important side-effects will become apparent. It is usually impracticable for the results of such multiple centre trials to be combined into one report and it is more valuable if each is designed to be statistically valid on its own. The results are therefore complementary, and if, for example, five different centres produce the same conclusion it is extremely unlikely that the drug has been incorrectly evaluated in any of them. This type of investigation will probably involve above 100 patients studied at five centres and will satisfy the criteria of different investigators, different centres, different patients and different conditions proposed by Lasagna (1955).

Stage 3

If the preliminary results obtained from Stage 1 and Stage 2 trials are satisfactory the drug should enter the final assessment of the Stage 3 trial. During this phase it will be given to a large number of patients over a prolonged period of perhaps one to two years. Particular attention will be paid to the correct dosage for the individual patient, to the development of side effects, and to comparison with other drugs having a similar action, Ideally the study will be planned so that the condition of patients is regularly assessed by an experienced clinician and 6-monthly assessment is satisfactory. At each visit a full history should be taken and clinical examination carried out including a 12 lead ECG. Particular attention should be paid to the development of tolerance to the drug. It is wise also to try to reduce the dosage from time to time in case the patient has improved spontaneously and an exaggerated impression of the efficacy of the drug is obtained.

The aims of such Stage 3 trials are (1) to evaluate the clinical value of the new product in relation to those already in use, (2) to attempt to determine how many patients will benefit from it, and (3) if it is suitable for any particular type of patient. It is important to realise that trials such as these are only meaningful if they are based upon the results of successful previous Stage 1 and Stage 2 investigations. Uncontrolled results obtained when a new drug is given casually to a few patients with angina over a relatively short period are of no value.

CHOICE OF END-POINT

The investigator is presented with a ' test system ' (i.e. the patient) in which various end-points can be chosen (Fig. 2).

Broadly speaking anti-anginal drugs may be evaluated according to two methods which are sometimes distinguished as ' subjective ' or ' objective '. The decision as to which type of method to employ must be taken at each Stage of the trial, 1, 2 or 3.

Subjective

Patients with angina present with the symptom of chest pain and the main aim of treatment (with anti-anginal drugs) is to give relief from that pain. This cannot be measured: it can only be assessed from the patient's (subjective) appreciation of his pain. Thus a patient's preference for one of two drugs is an acceptable and valid criterion of their relative efficacy.

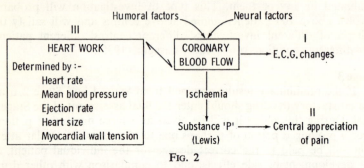

FIG. 2

' Test system ' for anti-anginal drugs. Numerals refer to parameters used to determine drug effects in angina. (Reproduced, with permission, from Fitzgerald, 1968.)

Objective

The so-called objective method depends on measurement of the alteration in exercise tolerance or perhaps on comparison of ECG changes of ischaemia developing at similar times during repeated exercise tests with and without the trial drug (Fig. 3). Both variants involve acute tests and are not readily applicable to patients in their everyday life.

In fact, measurement of exercise tolerance depends upon the patient's subjective decision when he has reached his limit of effort. To that extent this method also is subjective, although the results can usually be more readily analysed statistically and may be more repeatable than those obtained merely by questioning the patient.

On the other hand, a test of a drug's capacity to affect ECG changes is not a test of its effect on anginal pain. It is implied that the effects on the ECG relate to an effect on myocardial oxygenation, but this is seldom proved. However, the capacity of a drug to reduce or prevent ECG changes of ischaemia is obviously a measure of drug effect and usually, but not always, parallels its effect in relieving anginal pain.

In theory it is possible for the ECG changes to be used as a completely objective measurement since the exercise test could be stopped when the same degree of ST segment or T wave alteration has been reached during two exercise tests; this method would thus provide a more accurate and a safer end-point than relying upon the patient's subjective decision. In practice, it is quite impossible to achieve this ideal since firstly, the ECG changes usually progress even if the exercise is stopped, secondly it is not practicable for the investigator to quantitate changes in the ECG rapidly and accurately enough,

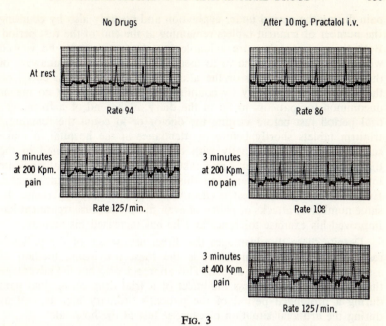

FIG. 3

ECGs taken during exercise before and after 10 mg Practolol given intra-venously at 300 kpm/min. After the drug the heart rate was slower, the ECG shows less ST segment depression and the patient had no anginal pain.

and thirdly the **type** of change may be different after the drug. It is not possible for an observer to judge accurately, for example, whether steep T wave inversion at a slow heart rate on the post-drug exercise test is equivalent to ST segment depression without T wave changes but occurring at a fast heart rate during the original control run. Even if the investigator were capable of this feat, the assessment would still be subjective. The ECG is usually displayed on an oscilloscope whereas it would be necessary to have a computer with continuous data comparison if ECG changes were to be used for determination of the end-point.

The usual method of analysis is a *subjective* assessment by the investigator at the end of the investigation of the ECGs recorded during the exercise test. It is therefore possible for comparisons to be made of the degree of ST segment depression or T wave inversion at the same exercise level before and after the drug. This is a useful but retrospective piece of information in deciding the effectiveness of an anti-anginal agent.

Combination of both methods

It may be possible to obtain additional data by asking patients to fill in a diary noting the frequency, character and duration of anginal pain during the period under evaluation and possibly also by counting the number of trinitrin tablets remaining at the end of the rest period. Both these approaches are valuable but the results must be viewed with caution since it is naïve to assume that patients are unaware of the purpose of the diary or the attempts by the doctor to check on the accuracy of the story by counting the tablets. It is by no means uncommon for patients to fill in the diary at the end of a fortnight's trial period just before visiting the doctor or to count the remaining trinitrin tablets shortly before re-attendance at the hospital to make sure that they check exactly with the attacks of pain noted in the diary. Furthermore, patients may take trinitrin prophylactically despite instructions to the contrary and this renders tablet counting invalid. Even if the drug under test is effective the patient may experience the same number of attacks of pain—or even more—because treatment has improved his exercise tolerance and he has increased his activity.

Despite these disadvantages the direct assessment of the patient's response to an unknown tablet is the most convincing method of assessing the *symptom* of angina. This approach also has the advantage that it is possible to assess the effect of a trial drug on anginal pain during a prolonged period of the patient's ordinary life, as well as during the artificial situation of exercise test at the hospital.

MODE OF ACTION STUDIES

There are two mechanisms by which drugs can relieve or prevent anginal pain.

1. They can allow the heart to perform more work, before pain is experienced.

2. They can allow the patient to perform more work without reaching the level of cardiac work at which pain is experienced.

In the first mode of action 'angina threshold' of the heart is actually increased but in the second this is not so. The ratio cardiac work/total body work is altered and there need be no effect on the maximum ability of the heart. It is likely that a drug working through the first mechanism will have a direct influence on cardiac muscle, but drugs acting through the second mechanism need not affect the heart directly since they might act through purely peripheral mechanisms (Fig. 4). It is of interest that all anti-anginal drugs known today appear to act through the second mechanism and no compound has been discovered which increases the ability of the heart to perform work beyond the point at which pain is felt.

It is conceivable that long term administration of anti-anginal drugs might increase the coronary blood flow in existing vessels or accelerate new vessel formation, but there is no reliable data that either of these mechanisms is clinically important with existing compounds.

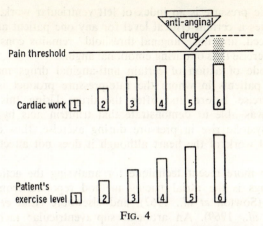

Fig. 4

Diagrammatic representation of two possible modes
of action of anti-anginal drugs. As the patient
increases his level of exercise the cardiac work
increases correspondingly until anginal pain is
produced at 'level 5'. An anti-anginal drug allows
the patient to exercise at 'level 6' without pain
either by increasing the pain threshold (dotted line)
to allow cardiac work to increase, *or* by reducing
cardiac work below the pain threshold.

Angina threshold

The usual explanation for the development of anginal pain is that
the myocardial oxygen demand has just exceeded the ability of the
coronary arteries to supply oxygen. The work of the heart and hence
the oxygen consumption depends upon many factors of which the
main ones are the tension developed in the ventricular muscle during
systole, the rate of contraction of the cardiac muscle, and the
heart rate. The myocardial wall tension is dependent upon the size
of the heart and the LV systolic pressure, the relationship being given
by 'La Place's Equation' (Levine and Wagman, 1962). This can be
stated most simply in the form

$$\text{Tension} = \alpha \, \frac{\text{pressure} \times \text{radius}}{2}$$

It is apparent that if the radius and therefore the heart size are small,
the wall tension and therefore the myocardial oxygen uptake will be
low for any given blood pressure. Similarly, if the blood pressure is
lowered, even with the heart remaining the same size, the wall tension
and myocardial oxygen uptake will be reduced.

In clinical terms it is difficult to measure myocardial wall tension,
but the inter-relationship of this with other factors allows conclusions
to be drawn from simple measurements of blood pressure and ejection
time. Robinson (1967) has shown that if the heart size and ejection
time remain fairly constant then the product of the heart rate and

peak systolic pressure is an index of left ventricular work. When this index reaches a certain critical level for any one patient anginal pain is experienced, and this 'anginal threshold' remains constant during repeated exercise tests or during emotional angina.

The mode of action of certain anti-anginal drugs may thus be studied in patients in whom the rate-pressure product is measured during exercise before and after the drug. Using this technique Robinson was able to demonstrate that trinitrin acts by preventing the usual systolic rise in pressure during exercise, thus diminishing the external work of the heart although it does not affect heart rate greatly.

Another more recent technique for analysing the action of anti-anginal drugs is the atrial pacing method reported from our own laboratory (Sowton et al., 1967), and elsewhere (Lau et al., 1967; Linhart et al., 1969). An artificial supraventricular tachycardia is produced by pacing the right atrium electrically and the heart rate increased by increments of 10 beats/min. until very mild angina is experienced. The pain can be immediately relieved if the heart rate is again reduced and the results are highly reproducible in most patients. The technique increased the myocardial oxygen demand through its effect on heart rate and we have shown that the 'angina threshold' can be accurately determined in terms of the tension time index (Sowton et al., 1967). This index has been shown in animals to relate to the myocardial oxygen uptake and is very similar to the rate-pressure product used by Robinson. Comparison between the 'angina threshold' measured by atrial pacing and by exercise-induced angina showed that the levels were extremely similar confirming that valid clinical judgements can be made on the basis of the test (Fig. 5).

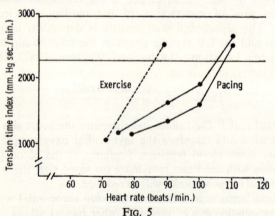

FIG. 5

The angina threshold expressed in terms of the tension-time index, was very similar when pain was induced by pacing or by exercise. (Reproduced by permission from Balcon et al., 1969.)

Using this technique it is possible to measure the 'angina threshold' three times and then to repeat the measurements after an anti-anginal drug has been given. Effects on myocardial contractility, peripheral circulatory response, or ejection rate may thus be studied although the technique is obviously not suitable for assessing drugs whose primary mode of action is by slowing the heart rate during exercise. It does however allow even these drugs to be studied with the object of determining whether there is any other action apart from brady-cardia. Studies already performed confirm that the action of trinitrin is peripheral rather than central (Frick *et al.*, 1968) and that the anti-anginal effect of propranolol is largely due to its rate effect (Balcon *et al.*, 1970).

An even more elaborate technique is described (Gorlin *et al.*, 1959; Gorlin, 1962) where simultaneous measurements are made of coronary blood flow by Krypton washout and haemodynamics by measuring left ventricular, brachial artery and coronary sinus pressure, together with arterial and coronary venous oxygen and lactate concentrations. In addition, left ventricular volume is measured by thermodilution and end-diastolic volume by a cineventriculographic method. With such a technique, it is possible to derive correlations for the effect of the drug on myocardial oxygen consumption, heart work and blood flow. It should be noted that coronary cine-angiography by itself shows *only* vessel diameter without any relation to total blood flow.

There are many other possible mechanisms by which anti-anginal drugs might influence cardiac metabolism, for example by inhibition of phosphorylation (Honig *et al.*, 1960), or by blocking of a possible 'oxygen-wasting' effect of catecholamines as suggested by Raab and Lepeschkin (1950) and by Raab (1962).

SUMMARY AND CONCLUSIONS

New anti-anginal drugs can satisfactorily be evaluated in three stages. Initially they are studied with a single blind technique in a few patients during acute experiments. Secondly, double blind cross-over trials with oral administration in a moderate number of patients are carried out, and lastly long term evaluation with optimal dosage in large numbers of patients for several years are needed.

Studies of the mode of action of effective drugs can be initiated with simple haemodynamic measurements and expanded to more complex metabolic studies.

Since angina is a symptom it is usually impossible to avoid a subjective element in drug evaluation either on the part of the patient or the investigator. Nevertheless repeatable results can be obtained and a statistical evaluation carried out. The final place of the drug in clinical practice cannot be determined until it has been compared with existing preparations over several years.

REFERENCES

ARMITAGE, P. (1954). Sequential tests in prophylactic and therapeutic trials. *Q. J. Med.* **23**, 255.

BALCON, R., BARCELO, J., HOY, J. & SOWTON, G. E. (1970). Rate-independent effects of propranolol and I.C.I. 50172 studies by atrial pacing. In press.

BATTERMAN, R. C. & GROSSMAN, A. J. (1955). Effectiveness of Salicylamide as an analgesic and anti-rheumatic agent. *J. Am. med. Ass.* **159**, 17.

BEECHER, H. K. (1955). The powerful placebo. *J. Am. med. Ass.* **159**, 1602.

BURKHART, F., BAROLD, S. & SOWTON, G. E. (1967). Haemodynamic effects of repeated exercise. *Am. J. Cardiol.* **20**, 509.

CHAMBERLAIN, D. A. (1966). The haemodynamic effects of beta adrenergic blockade in man. *Cardiolog.* **49**, Suppl. 2, 27.

COLE, S. A. & GRIFFITH, G. C. (1958). Assay of anti-anginal agents; the Rapport period. *J. Am. med. Ass.* **168**, 275.

CONWAY, N., GUPTA, G. D. & SOWTON, G. E. (1968). Failure of Intensain to improve exercise tolerance in patients with angina pectoris. *Acta cardiol.* **23**, 434.

EVANS, W. & HOYLE, C. (1933). The comparative value of drugs used in the continuous treatment of angina pectoris. *Q. J. Med.* **2**, 311.

FITZGERALD, J. D. (1968). Testing of anti-anginal drugs. In *Testing Methods of Vasoactive Drug Effects*. Ed. Becattini, U. Rome: C.E.P.I.

FRICK, M. J., BALCON, R., CROSS, D. & SOWTON, G. E. (1968). Haemodynamic effects of nitroglycerine in patients with angina pectoris studied by an atrial pacing method. *Circulation* **37**, 160.

GIBSON, D., HOY, J. & SOWTON, G. E. (1970). Comparison between oxprenolol and alprenolol during steady state exercise. In press.

GORLIN, R. (1962). Drugs and angina pectoris. *Am. J. Cardiol.* 19, 419.

GORLIN, R., BRACHFIELD, N., MACLED, C. & BOPP, P. (1959). Effect of nitroglycerin on the pulmonary and systemic circulation in patients with increased left ventricular work. *Circulation,* **19**, 705.

HONIG, C. R., TENSEY, S. M. & GABLE, P. V. (1960). The mechanism of cardio-vascular action of nitroglycerine. *Am. J. Med.* **29**, 910.

LASAGNA, L. (1955). The controlled clinical trial—theory and practice. *J. chron. Dis.* **1**, 353.

LAU, S., HAFT, J., COHEN, S., KINNEY, M., HELFANT, R., YOUNG, M. & DAMATO, A. (1967). Controlled heart rates in the evaluation of angina pectoris. *Clin. Res.* **15**, 212.

LEVINE, H. J. & WAGMAN, R. J. (1962). Energetics of the human heart. *Am. J. Cardiol.* **8**, 772.

LINHART, J. W., HILDEN, F. J., BAROLD, S. S., LISTER, J. W. & SAMET, P. (1969). Left heart haemodynamics during angina pectoris induced by atrial pacing. *Am. J. Cardiol.* **23**, 124.

RAAB, W. (1962). The sympathogenic biochemical trigger mechanism of angina pectoris. *Am. J. Cardiol.* **8**, 576.

RAAB, W. & LEPSECHKIN, E. (1950). The anti-adrenergic effects of nitroglycerine on the heart. *Circulation,* **1**, 733.

ROBINSON, B. F. (1967). Relation of heart rate and systolic blood pressure to the onset of pain in angina pectoris. *Circulation,* **35**, 1073.

SOWTON, G. E., BALCON, R., CROSS, D. & FRICK, M. H. (1967). Measurements of the angina threshold using atrial pacing. *Cardiovasc. Res.* **1**, No. 4, 301.

SOWTON, G. E. & BURKHART, F. (1967). Haemodynamic changes during continuous exercise. *Br. Heart J.* **29**, 770.

THE EVALUATION OF LIPID LOWERING AGENTS

J. D. FITZGERALD

Introduction

Most people currently believe that an understanding of lipid pathophysiology will lead to an understanding of atherosclerosis, and this in turn will lead to the possibility of controlling the progress of atherosclerosis—a disease considered responsible for the majority of deaths in many parts of the world. However, we must bear in mind that a critical examination of the relationship between the level of serum lipids, the incidence of atherosclerosis and the incidence of the clinical syndromes of coronary artery disease and cerebral athero-sclerosis indicates certain discrepancies. Before discussing aspects of lipid control by pharmacological means, certain points must be kept in mind.

Atherosclerosis is a problem of extreme complexity in which diet, endocrine metabolism, enzyme systems, and other factors such as sex, heredity, environmental strain, smoking and physical activity may be involved. Thus atherosclerotic vascular disease may be viewed as the resultant of a number of environmental factors which act and interact with host factors in determining its origin, progress and final clinical manifestations. Any study which sets out to evaluate the effect of a particular intervention on this condition must bear in mind the multifactorial causation of the disease. However, it is worth emphasis-ing that the disease is not an inevitable consequence of ageing, and that its presence and severity differ widely from one population to another and between individuals within populations. Evaluating the contribution of each of the factors listed above is made more difficult because of one or more of the following factors:

1. The apparent complexity of the tissue and haemodynamic factors influencing the location and evolution of the atherosclerotic lesion

2. The still imperfectly understood relation between the underlying atherosclerotic lesion and the subsequent clinical syndrome

3. The inability to assess conveniently the presence and extent of atherosclerosis in vivo

4. The absence of an adequate experimental animal model for atherosclerosis.

CLINICAL SYNDROMES

By definition, atherosclerosis is a pathological condition and not a clinical syndrome. There may be a difference between showing that a particular intervention affects the course of a clinical syndrome and assuming that the *same* intervention affects the course of atherosclerosis.

A therapeutic agent which lowers the mortality in ischaemic heart disease may not necessarily affect the atherosclerotic process. However, our present view is that an agent which will affect the atherosclerotic process should secondarily diminish the incidence of the associated clinical syndromes. Though coronary atherosclerosis is universal in advanced countries, ischaemic heart disease is not. This observation leads to a consideration therefore of such factors predisposing towards the development of ischaemic heart disease. Numerous surveys have indicated that healthy individuals with some or all of the following characteristics will tend to have a greater incidence of ischaemic heart disease:

1. Hyperlipidaemic states
2. Essential hypertension
3. Cigarette smoking
4. Physical inactivity
5. Premature cessation of ovarian activity
6. Low vital capacity.

Such surveys include the results of the Cooperative Study (1956) and the Symposium (1957) as well as the work of Katz and Stamler (1958), Lee and Schneider (1958), Thomas (1958), Doyle et al. (1959), Stamler (1959), Zukel (1959), Berkson et al. (1960), Epstein (1960), the Metropolitan Life Insurance Company (1960), Stamler et al. (1960), Symposium (1960), Pell and D'Alonzo (1960; 1961), Spain (1961), Stamler et al. (1961), Gertler et al. (1969) and Paul et al. (1956).

Other important influences are diabetes, psychogenic stress and the reaction of the individual to it, a rapid gain in weight, hyperuricaemia and a thrombotic tendency.

HYPERLIPIDAEMIA AND ATHEROSCLEROSIS

The association of an accelerated development of both athero-sclerosis and coronary heart disease with disorders in which the levels of blood lipids are grossly elevated has long been recognised (De Langen, 1916; Katz and Stamler, 1953). However, it has only been in the last 15 years or so that prospective epidemiological studies have demonstrated the clear and quantitative association between the level of certain blood lipids and the subsequent incidence of coronary and thrombotic vascular disease. The full implications of this association are not agreed by all investigators in this field. Thus, Bronte-Stewart (1959), while admitting that certain diseases such as diabetes mellitus and essential xanthomatosis are associated with an increased tendency towards severe atherosclerosis and a higher incidence of ischaemic heart disease, suggests that much of the data relating ischaemic heart disease to a disorder of fat metabolism is based on associations and extrapolations which need not necessarily indicate causal connection. The association between hyperlipidaemia and ischaemic heart disease is based on four types of observation (Oliver,

1967b): that (1) arterial lesions contain lipid, (2) induced hyper-lipidaemia in animals leads to arterial lesions rich in lipids, (3) patients with the symptom complex of ischaemic heart disease often have abnormal serum lipid levels and (4) hypercholesterolaemia, at least, is associated with an increased risk of developing ischaemic heart disease.

Hyperlipidaemia is common in patients with ischaemic heart disease, especially in young patients. The Cooperative Study (1956) indicated that the concentration of all the major serum lipids, i.e. cholesterol, phospholipids and triglycerides, is elevated in subjects with coronary heart disease. Since virtually all serum lipids are present as lipoproteins, correlations have also been developed between the various lipoprotein classes and the incidence of coronary heart disease. There is no evidence that the chemical composition of the lipoprotein classes is altered substantially in subjects with coronary artery disease compared with normal persons. Therefore, measurement of either the serum lipoprotein or the serum lipids will reflect similar abnormalities. Because of the ease of estimating cholesterol, this has been the lipid that has been most extensively studied. Thus, the Framingham Study (Kagan *et al.*, 1963) showed that the risk of developing ischaemic heart disease may be increased as much as six times in subjects with hyper-cholesterolaemia compared with those with low plasma cholesterol levels. Similar findings have been reported by others (Carlson, 1960; Havel and Carlson, 1962; Brown *et al.*, 1965). On the other hand, Carlson's data suggest that the concentration of the S_f 20-400 lipo-proteins, which are relatively rich in triglycerides, correlates more closely with the presence of coronary heart disease than that of the S_f 0-12 lipoproteins which are relatively rich in cholesterol. Albrink's study (1961) of triglyceride levels, peripheral and coronary artery disease, confirmed this view, though Carlson's data suggests that it is only in people under the age of 50 that the triglyceride-coronary artery disease correlation is valid (Table I). It is clear that neither the estima-

TABLE I

*Comparison of Serum Triglyceride Concentration in Men Calculated from Data of Various Investigators**

Decade	Gofman (1954)		Carlson (1960)		Albrink (1961)	
	Control	Coronary	Control†	Coronary	Control	Coronary
4th	140	—	112	226	114	252
5th	136	186	112	190	138	189
6th	142	185	112	127	147	252
7th	133	145	112	131	138	198

* Values expressed as mg per 100 ml serum.
† 112 for middle-aged men; decades not specified.

(Reproduced with permission from Havel, R. J. & Carlson, L. A., 1962, *Metabolism*, **11**, 195.)

tion of cholesterol nor triglyceride *alone* gives an adequate picture of altered lipoprotein concentrations. Therefore, in assessing whether or not a patient has hyperlipidaemia, the serum cholesterol and serum triglyceride should be measured simultaneously and on several occasions. When this is done, it is possible to detect atherosclerotic patients with three characteristics:

1. Elevated concentrations of very low density lipoproteins (S_f 20-400) (predominantly hypertriglyceridaemia) with normal concentrations of low density lipoproteins (S_f 0-20) (predominantly cholesterol)

2. Elevated low density lipoproteins (S_f 0-20) (predominantly cholesterol) with normal very low density lipoproteins (predominantly triglycerides).

3. Elevation of both lipoprotein fractions, i.e. both cholesterol and triglyceride.

Recently, Thorp (Stone and Thorp, 1966) has developed a simplified method for determining the S_f 20-400 fraction by means of a simple micronephelometer. This instrument is used in combination with suitable filtration techniques and will enable one to determine (1) the degree of chylomicronaemia and (2) the extent of the S_f 20-400 class of lipoprotein. From these and a measurement of the serum cholesterol, it is possible to derive the extent of the S_f 0-20 lipoprotein class. Thus it is possible to obtain a complete and quantitative profile of the low density lipoproteins. The advantage of such a technique over both the non- quantitative electrophoretic method and the expensive time-consuming ultracentrifugal analysis is obvious (Fig. 1).

Diet and atherosclerosis

The evidence indicates that of the many factors involved in the pathogenesis of atherosclerosis, hyperlipidaemia is of over-riding importance. There is much evidence which relates nutrition to the progress of atherosclerotic vascular disease and to the clinical sequelae. Since dietary alterations can significantly influence blood lipids, nutrition is of importance in both the treatment of the disease and also in relation to assessing drugs which may have a hypolipidaemic effect. A recent review (McGandy et al., 1967) concluded that the only way in which diet may affect the development and progression of atherosclerosis is by influencing the level of serum lipids, especially serum cholesterol. There is no doubt that levels of serum cholesterol can be modified by alterations of both the levels of fat and cholesterol in the diet. The alterations that are most likely to cause a lowering of the serum cholesterol are (1) a lowering of the proportion of dietary saturated fatty acids (2) increasing the proportion of polyunsaturated fatty acids, and (3) reducing the level of dietary cholesterol.

In addition, there is evidence that both the kind and amount of dietary carbohydrate is important in the regulation of serum lipids.

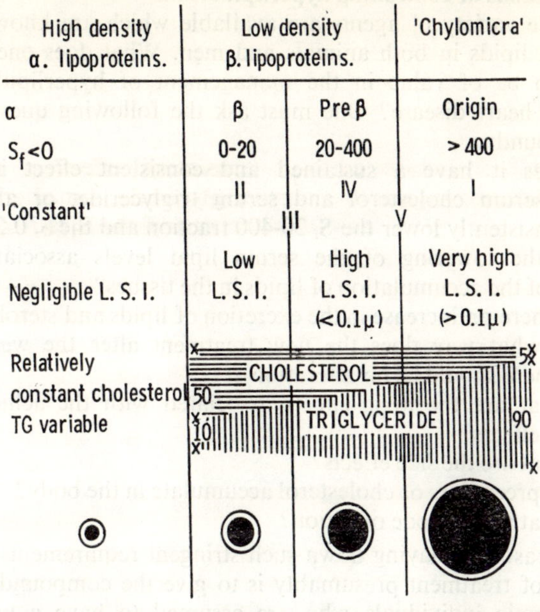

FIG. 1

(Lower half) Relationship between lipoprotein particle size, the cholesterol and triglyceride content. (Upper half) Relationship between electrophoretic mobility, lipoprotein density and light scattering properties of serum (L.S.I.). Also included is the Fredrickson classification Type I to Type V in terms of the dominant lipoprotein disturbance. Since the micronephelometer will determine both the chylomicra and the S_1 20-400 fraction, then if the serum cholesterol is known, a qualitative picture of the serum lipoproteins is obtained.

However, the importance of diet in reducing the *risk* of the clinical complications of atherosclerosis has yet to be established. Long-term clinical trials which meet the criteria outlined later are still needed to determine whether a reduction in serum cholesterol by altering the diet will in fact improve the morbidity and mortality rates. A recent report from the Anti-Coronary Club in New York (Christakis *et al.*, 1966) suggests that a significant reduction in the incidence of coronary heart disease in a group of men whose average level of serum cholesterol was reduced by 12 per cent on a diet restricted in saturated fats and cholesterol while increased in *polyunsaturated* fats resulted in a significant reduction in the incidence of coronary heart disease. A similar study (Leren, 1966) from Oslo also shows an encouraging improvement if the diet, similar to that used by the Anti-Coronary Club in New York, is utilised.

Other methods of controlling hyperlipidaemia

A wide variety of agents are available which are known to lower the serum lipids in both animals and men. What does one require of a drug to be of value in the management of hyperlipidaemia and ischaemic heart disease? One must ask the following questions about the compound:

1. Does it have a sustained and consistent effect in reducing elevated serum cholesterol and serum triglyceride, or alternatively, does it consistently lower the S_f 20-400 fraction and the S_f 0-20 fraction?

2. Is the lowering of the serum lipid levels associated with a lowering of the accumulation of lipids in the tissues?

3. Is there an increase in the excretion of lipids and sterols?

4. In what way does the new treatment alter the way of living (ideally, there should be no alteration)?

5. What are the toxic effects associated with the achievement of the above effects?

6. What are the side effects?

7. Do precursors of cholesterol accumulate in the body?

8. What is the mode of action?

The reason for laying down such stringent requirements is that the final aim of treatment presumably is to give the compound to healthy hyperlipaemic individuals who are assumed to have a greater than usual risk of developing vascular disease and who may therefore need to take the drug for the rest of their lives. The fact that such prolonged treatment is necessary makes the use of a tablet or capsule much more attractive as a means of reducing elevated lipids than restricting the diet in one form or another. Whether atherosclerosis is the result of an abnormal lipid metabolic process may be controversial, but if a drug treatment could prevent the development of this disease and extend the life of the patients, no further justification would be needed in trying to develop an ideal anti-hyperlipaemic agent.

THE DESIGN OF TRIALS FOR HYPERLIPIDAEMIC AGENTS

AIMS OF TRIALS

These fall into three groups chronologically (Table II). The initial group of trials should aim to answer the following questions:

1. Does the lipid lowering agent lower elevated serum lipids to normal?

2. Is the effect consistent and persistent?

3. Does it affect thrombogenic mechanisms?

4. What are the toxic and side effects?

The second group of studies is concerned with the pharmacodynamics and mode of action of the hypolipidaemic agent and the final group is concerned with the morbidity and mortality studies to demonstrate that chronic lowering of lipids will diminish the incidence of clinical syndromes associated with atherosclerosis.

TABLE II

Summary of the Procedure for the Evaluation of a Hypolipidaemic Agent

GROUP A STUDIES

STUDIES TO DETERMINE THE EFFECT ON SERUM LIPIDS AND LIPOPROTEINS

Objectives:

1. What serum lipids does it affect?
2. What is the degree of hypolipidaemic activity?
3. Does the effect last as long as treatment continues?
4. What is the effect on thrombogenic mechanisms?
5. What are the side effects?

Other considerations:

1. Patient selection—age, sex, diet, weight, lipid levels and lipoprotein classification, other diseases (diabetes, gout, pregnancy, recent myocardial infarction)
2. Trial design
3. Trial duration
4. Organ toxicity
5. Criteria of effectiveness

GROUP B STUDIES

Objectives:

1. To characterise the absorption, distribution metabolism and excretion of the drug
2. To determine the mode of action

Other considerations:

1. Optimal blood level in relation to activity
2. Optimal dose required
3. Half-life (a) pharmacological; (b) chemical
4. Urine, biliary and faecal excretion

GROUP C STUDIES

Objective:

To determine the effect of chronic administration of the drug on morbidity and mortality

Other considerations:

1. Patient selection (a) high risk subjects; (b) subjects with clinical cardiovascular disease
2. Assessment—medical, social, family history, physical examination, ECG, lipid levels
3. Number of patients
4. Trial design. Simultaneously randomised double-blind study
5. Diet and weight
6. Follow-up

GROUP A TRIALS

The object of the trials is to demonstrate the hypolipidaemic action of the drug.

Patient selection

In selecting patients for study, the following factors are of importance:

Age and sex. Several workers have described a lowering in lipoprotein and cholesterol values in the very old person. The reason for this is not clear but must be taken into account in selecting patients for study. Similarly, it is known that in males there is a marked rise in beta-lipoprotein fraction of the serum as well as the total lipoprotein cholesterol during the third and fourth decade (Table I). On the other hand, females of the same age show a much smaller increase in these fractions and it is only when the post-menopausal era is reached that serum levels reach the equivalent level in the male. In addition, serum cholesterol and phospholipid concentrations undergo regular cyclic changes in the female (Oliver and Boyd, 1953). At the mid-point of the menstrual cycle, there is a decline in total cholesterol, as well as a drop in cholesterol phospholipid ratio. During the follicular and luteal phases of the cycle, there is a greater increase in the circulating cholesterol than in phospholipids, thus elevating the ratio. Furthermore, there is also a seasonal variation in cholesterol levels.

Diet and weight. Reference has already been made to the profound influence of the effects of diet on serum lipids. Thus not only is the total caloric intake important, but also the qualitative nature of the diet, particularly in regard to the content of polyunsaturated fatty acids, the amount of cholesterol in the diet and the kind and amount of dietary carbohydrate. Furthermore a positive correlation has been shown between relative body weight and the concentration of plasma triglycerides. Patients who are overweight tend to have increased triglyceride levels (Sailer *et al.*, 1966). When a patient is admitted to a trial, it is imporant that his weight is measured during the duration of the trial to determine the possible influence of this on the lipid response. Therefore, the patient must be instructed to maintain himself within reasonably narrow limits of the type of food that he has been taking for the previous few months and to maintain the same degree of caloric intake with little fluctuation in body weight.

Other diseases. It is important to exclude patients from this study who have diabetes mellitus, gout, a recent myocardial infarct or pregnancy. The serum lipids in these conditions can alter profoundly without any pharmacological intervention.

Lipid levels. The criterion for admission to a trial will clearly be elevation of the lipid levels. However, it is still a matter of controversy as to what constitutes a normal serum lipid level and furthermore, which lipids should be measured. The very low density and the low density lipoproteins should be estimated, directly if possible. If this is not possible, then the serum cholesterol and the serum triglycerides must be measured at the same time. The timing of the taking of the blood sample is important. The patient should be fasting for the previous 12 to 14 hours, and should not have had an excess of alcohol in the previous 24 hours. If possible, blood should be taken at about the same time of the day on each occasion.

The newborn child has a plasma cholesterol of approximately 75 to 100 ml. It may well be that a normal adult level should be moderately above this. The Institute for Metabolic Research in the United States have placed the upper limits of normal for cholesterol at 180 mg, for phospholipids at 200 mg and for triglycerides at approximately 100 mg. However, in addition to the absolute lipid measurement, the classification of lipid disorder is important. Most investigators would now agree that the Fredrickson classification has brought a great deal of clarity to a rather confused field. Any patient in future who is being considered for a trial of a hypolipidaemic agent should have his lipoprotein pattern classified. If this is not done, it may well be that an agent which is effective in a certain type of hyperlipidaemia, but not in another type, may be rejected because the patients selected for study have a hyperlipidaemia of the resistant type. Of course it is equally important to ensure that at some point in the studies, *all* of the Fredrickson types of hyperlipidaemia are subjected to study.

Trials design. In the initial application of the drug to the human, it is necessary of course to use an open therapeutic design in order that no untoward event may take place. However, having shown in a preliminary study that the agent appears to lower serum lipids, it is necessary to alter the design of the study to a double-blind cross-over type. Quite remarkable objective and subjective responses can be obtained in patients receiving placebos and it is therefore necessary to ensure that the hypolipidaemic response is in fact due to the administration of the active compound and not due to increased care and attention on the part of the doctor and the other many factors that alter the environment of the patient once he is admitted to a clinical trial.

Duration. The duration of this initial study will depend on the mode of action and degree of activity of the hypolipidaemic agent. Certainly it is important to demonstrate *not only* that serum lipids can be lowered initially, but that this initial lowering is maintained over a significant period of time and I would suggest a period of 6 to 9 months as a minimum. Clofibrate, for example, clearly fulfils this requirement.

Organ toxicity. During this period of observation, important data should be collected on the effect of the drug on various organs. It is essential, therefore, that routine liver function tests, renal function tests, and assessment of the circulating elements in the blood is made.

Criteria for effectiveness. Serum lipids should be measured at weekly intervals initially for a period of four weeks, then at fortnightly intervals for a further four weeks and then at monthly intervals for the duration of the trial. The effectiveness of the agent can be described in terms either of the percentage fall related to the baseline lipid levels, or alternatively, to the number of patients who attain and maintain normal lipid levels.

GROUP B TRIALS

These trials are concerned with the pharmacodynamics of the hypo-lipidaemic agent and its mode of action. Naturally they will tend to overlap with the Group A trials but are unlikely to be carried out in any detail unless a hypolipidaemic action has already been demonstrated in the human.

Pharmacodynamic studies

These will be of the classical kind concerned with the determination of the oral dose necessary to give optimal blood levels and these should be related to the blood levels required to lower the elevated serum lipids in animals and man. In addition, studies should be carried out to determine the effect of the compound on organ function and also to determine its metabolism, distribution and excretion.

Mode of action studies

The nature of the studies on the mode of action of the compound in the human will be governed to a large extent by the findings in animal studies. If the compound works, for example, by inhibiting cholesterol and fat absorption in animals, then clearly studies in the human will be orientated to determine the effect of the compound on the absorption of vitamins, minerals and other food stuffs. Information of fat excretion, calcium absorption, serum levels of electrolytes, the absorption of vitamins A and D during drug treatment, etc. will be necessary. Furthermore, studies to determine its effect on the long-term nutritional status of the patient are essential.

If the drug acts by inhibiting cholesterol and triglyceride synthesis, then attention should be directed to the tissue and serum levels of cholesterol precursors, particularly those on the biosynthetic pathway between mevalonic acid and cholesterol. Therefore, analysis of human serum by appropriate techniques such as thin layer chromatographic separation of the unsaponifiable fractions is necessary. Frequently the serum levels will reflect what is occurring in the tissues. Estimation of the level of cholesterol precursors in a tissue such as the skin is desirable, if this is feasible. Of more importance is the level of the lipids in the tissues, especially triglycerides and cholesterol. Thus both thyroxine and d-thyroxine elevate the total body cholesterol in rats during treatment even though the serum levels of cholesterol are lower than in the control group (Duncan *et al.*, 1964). On the other hand, clofibrate lowers both total body cholesterol and the serum levels (Nestel *et al.*, 1965). In essence, it must be shown that a hypolipidaemic agent does not lower serum lipids by merely redistributing the total body lipids. Similarly, studies to determine the rate of incorporation of radio-labelled cholesterol precursors should be done, as well as studies to determine the effect of the drug on the total body pool of cholesterol. It is also necessary to determine the effect of the agent on the faecal excretion of sterols which should increase if the agent is enhancing cholesterol excretion. In the case of clofibrate, it has been shown that the total body pool can be diminished and faecal sterol excretion increased without any change in serum cholesterol (Oliver, 1967b).

GROUP C TRIALS

These trials are concerned with answering the most important question of all: does the administration of the hypolipidaemic drug bring about a diminution in the morbidity and mortality of the clinical syndromes associated with atherosclerosis? The complementary question is: does it reduce the degree of arterial atherosclerosis? Studies designed to answer these questions will be large, lengthy, detailed, time-consuming, and very expensive. Let us consider firstly studies designed to reduce the morbidity and mortality.

What sort of subjects are suitable for inclusion in the study? They fall into two basic types. Firstly the subject that has already presented clinically with one of the syndromes of atherosclerosis, most commonly myocardial infarction or angina pectoris. The advantage of choosing such a type is that one is certain that the subject has an important degree of atherosclerosis and also, one can estimate roughly the mortality and morbidity of such a group of subjects from the abundant data on the natural history of the condition. However, there are difficulties even here. For once a patient has been selected for a clinical study, he is not exactly the same person any more, and one cannot always assume that one's selected group will behave predictably. Certainly the mortality from coronary artery disease varies very considerably, even in adjacent countries, if one is to judge from the results of comparative studies in these countries.

Another objection to choosing such subjects is that the atherosclerotic process may be too far advanced for any form of therapy to reverse the process. However, we do know from experimental studies in rats with calcified aortic disease, that clofibrate can reverse the lesions in 6 to 12 months. I would emphasise that these are naturally occurring lesions and not induced by dietary manipulation. In addition to these objections is the fact that many other factors apart from hyperlipidaemia may play an important part in morbidity and mortality in such subjects.

The second approach is to select subjects who, whilst not manifesting clinical signs and symptoms of atherosclerosis, are nevertheless ' high risk ' subjects. Such studies are concerned with preventing the *initial* episode rather than *subsequent* episodes. It has been shown repeatedly that hyperlipidaemia, hypertension, smoking, obesity and certain ECG abnormalities are associated with significant increases in the risk of mortality and morbidity from coronary artery disease, especially when these factors are present in combination.

One may therefore select such subjects and administer the hypo-lipidaemic agent *prophylactically*. It must be explained to these subjects that: (1) they will be under medical supervision for three to five years, (2) they will have to have regular check-ups, (3) they will have to have blood samples taken and (4) they will have to consume X number of pills daily for this period and that there is a 50:50 chance that they are taking a placebo!

Assessment

Whichever type of subject is selected, the crucial point is the completeness and duration of the assessment and the quality of the follow-up. The following points must be elucidated in detail:

Social history
> Sex, age, marital status
> Occupation; social status, educational standard
> Smoking: how much, how long, if stopped, when?

Medical history
> Pain on effort: degree, frequency, precipitating factors
> Dyspnoea: degree
> Intermittent claudication
> Other pain of possibly ischaemic origin.

Previous history
> Relevant details are recorded.

Family history
> Especially (1) diabetes mellitus, (2) cerebro-vascular accident; (3) angina or coronary thrombosis and (4) cause of death.

Physical examination
> Especially blood pressure, cardiac murmurs, skinfold thickness —xanthomata.

Investigations
> Serum cholesterol and triglyceride levels (S_f 0-20 and 20-400 levels)
> ECG: These should be read by two independent observers and reported on in an agreed standard manner.

Other considerations in large scale prospective studies

The number of patients. In setting up such a prospective study, the first requirement is to know the number of patients and the duration of treatment required to give a significant result to the study. If it is assumed that the treatment is expected to reduce morbidity from, for example, 10 to 5 per cent per year, and mortality from 6 to 4 per cent per year, as a desirable minimal effect and if in addition it is necessary to demonstrate such a response with a significant $P=0.05$, then it is possible to calculate the number of patient/years of treatment required. If one wishes to have a 90 per cent confidence of the significance of the reduction in morbidity then 500 patient/years is required and 2,000 patient/years to be equally certain of a significant reduction in mortality. On the other hand, these numbers can be reduced to 200 and 750 patient/years respectively if you wish to lower the confidence limits to 50, rather than 90 per cent. There will, of course, be an equal number of patients in the placebo group. Therefore in such a study, the minimum number of patients would be, for morbidity 120, and for mortality 500. These should be studied for three years. However, in order to ensure that a result is obtained, far more patients are necessary to make allowance for patients who drop out of the trial, patients who have a delayed onset in response to treatment and patients who are not responders in the sense of a lipid response.

Diet and weight. In such a prospective study, it is essential to keep an accurate record of the weight of the patient during the whole period of the study. In addition, a clear idea as to any fundamental alteration in his diet should be obtained. In many published studies, particularly on the effect of unsaturated fats on morbidity and mortality, these aspects have been omitted. Information should be as accurate as possible concerning the adherence to diets in both the control and the treated group, as well as information on the contents of the diets.

Lipid measurements. Even though such studies would be on a massive scale, since the rationale behind them is to demonstrate that control of serum lipids will materially affect both morbidity and mortality, it is very desirable that repeated measurements of the serum cholesterol and triglyceride, or preferably the lipoprotein classes, should be carried out. It should be emphasised that adequate pre-treatment control levels must be obtained. It should be appreciated that the more heterogeneous a population, the less is the chance of obtaining a clear result.

Trial design. It is essential in any such prospective study that the trial should be a simultaneously randomised double-blind study of even numbered groups. If the numbers are large enough, the group will match. It is in this area that the greatest criticism has been placed in the past on clinical studies concerning the effects of both hypo-lipidaemic agents and low fat diets on morbidity and mortality. Thus the groups must be matched for age, sex, social status, educational status, religion and concomitant disease.

Follow-up. This must be complete. The fate of all patients in the trial should be known, the reason for any drop out, the cause of death and the pathology of the cardiovascular system.

From these remarks it is clear that any prospective study designed to determine the effect of the control of hyperlipidaemia in, for example, ischaemic heart disease is extremely difficult in terms of patient selection, the duration of the study, the control of the study and the cost of the study.

CONCLUSION

In this paper, I have attempted to summarise firstly the rationale for hypolipidaemic therapy in clinical medicine. Whilst there is evidence that hyperlipidaemia is of overriding importance in the pathogenesis of atherosclerosis and the concomitant diseases, it is as well to bear in mind constantly that several other factors are important and that in the individual case, they may be even more important than the serum lipid levels. Furthermore, it has yet to be shown that lowering serum lipid levels over a prolonged period of time materially affects the prognosis for life or morbidity in a given population. The control of lipids by dietary manipulation are sufficiently encouraging to justify the therapeutic approach to atherosclerosis by means of lowering serum lipids. The evaluation of a hypolipidaemic agent is a lengthy and meticulous matter. It involves the close collaboration between the clinician, biochemist, the epidemiologist and the biologist as well as the cooperation of the patient. In the present state of knowledge, it is not sufficient to demonstrate that an agent lowers serum lipids effectively and continuously. It is also required to prove that such a control will improve the morbidity and mortality of the diseases associated with atherosclerosis.

ACKNOWLEDGEMENT

I would like to thank my colleagues, Dr C. C. Downie and Mr J. M. Thorp, for their advice and criticism in the preparation of this paper, and Verlag Hans Huber Bern for permission to reproduce this paper.

REFERENCES

ALBRINK, M. J. (1961). Serum lipids, hypertension and coronary heart disease. Am. J. Med. 31, 4.

BERKSON, D. M., STAMLER, J., LINDBERG, H. A., MILLER, W., MATHIES, H., LASKY, H. & HALL, Y. (1960). Socioeconomic correlates of atherosclerotic and hypertensive heart disease. Proc. N.Y. Acad. Sci. 84, 835.

BRONTE-STEWART, B. (1959). Post-grad. med. J. 35, 198.

BROWN, D. F., KINCH, S. H. & DOYLE, J .T. (1965). Serum triglycerides in health and ischaemic heart disease. New Engl. J. Med. 237, 947.

CARLSON, L. A. (1960). Serum lipids in men with myocardial infarction. Acta med. scand. 167, 399.

CHRISTAKIS, G., RINZLER, S. H. & ARCHER, M. (1966). The Anti-coronary Club. A dietary approach to the prevention of coronary heart disease—a seven-year report. Am. J. publ. Hlth, 56, 299.

COOPERATIVE STUDY, (1956). Evaluation of serum lipoprotein and cholesterol measurements as predictors of clinical complications of atherosclerosis. Report of a cooperative study of lipoproteins and atherosclerosis. (20 authors). Circulation, 14, No. 4, Part 2.

DE LANGEN, C. O. (1916). Cholesterol metabolism and racial pathology. *Geneesk Tijdschr. Ned.-Indie,* **56,** 1.

DOYLE, J. T., HESLIN, A. S., HILLEBOE, H. E. & FORMEL, P. F. (1959). Early diagnosis of ischaemic heart disease. *New Engl. J. Med.* **261,** 1096.

DUNCAN, C. H., BEST, M. M. & LUBBE, R. J. (1964). Effects of l- and d-thyroxine and of thyroidectomy on tissue weights and cholesterol content of the rat. *Metabolism,* **13,** 1.

EPSTEIN, F. H. (1960). Epidemiology of coronary heart disease. *Modern Trends in Cardiology,* p. 155. London: Butterworth.

GERTLER, M. M., WOODBURY, M. A., GOTTSCH, L. G., WHITE, P. D. & RUSK, H. A. (1969). The candidate for coronary heart disease. Discriminating power of biochemical hereditary and anthropometric measurements. *J. Am. med. Ass.* **170,** 149.

HAVEL, R. J. & CARLSON, L. A. (1962). Serum lipid proteins, cholesterol and triglyceride in coronary heart disease. *Metabolism,* **11,** 195.

KAGAN, A., KANNEL, W. B. & DAWBER, T. R. (1963). The coronary profile. *Ann. N.Y. Acad. Sci.* **97,** 883.

KATZ, L. N. & STAMLER, J. (1953). *Experimental Atherosclerosis.* Springfield, Illinois: Thomas.

KATZ, L. N. & STAMLER, J. (1958). *Nutrition and Atherosclerosis.* Philadelphia: Lea and Febiger.

LEE, R. E. & SCHNEIDER, R. F. (1958). Hypertension and atherosclerosis in executive and nonexecutive personnel. *J. Am. med. Ass.* **167,** 1447.

LEREN, P. (1966). The effects of plasma cholesterol lowering diet in male survivors of myocardial infarction. *Norwegian Monographs on Medical Science,* Universitetsforlaget.

MCGANDY, R. B., HEGSTED, D. M. & STARE, F. J. (1967). Dietary fats, carbohydrates and atherosclerotic vascular disease. *New Engl. J. Med.* **277,** 186.

METROPOLITAN LIFE INSURANCE COMPANY (1960). Overweight, its prevention and significance. *Reprinted from Statistical Bulletin.* New York, N.Y.

MOSES, C. (1963). *Atherosclerosis.* London: Kimpton.

NESTEL, P. J., HIRSCH, E. Z., & COUZENS, E. A. (1965). The effect of chlorphenoxyisobutyric acid and ethinyl estradiol on cholesterol turnover. *J. clin. Invest.* **44,** 891.

OLIVER, M. F. & BOYD, G. S. (1953). Changes in plasma lipids during menstrual cycle. *Clin. Sci.* **12,** 217.

OLIVER, M. F. (1967a). Editorial, The present status of Clofibrate (Atromid-S). *Circulation,* **36,** 337.

OLIVER, M. F. (1967b). In *Recent Advances in Pharmacology and Therapeutics,* p. 221. ed. Fulton, W. F. M. London: Butterworth.

PAUL, D., OSTFELD, A. M. & LEPPER, M. H. (1956). *An Anterospective Study of Coronary Heart Disease.* Privately printed.

PAUL, O., LEPPER, M. H., PHELAN, W. H., DUPERTUIS, G. W., MACMILLAN, A., MCKEAN, H. & PARK, H. (1963). A longitudinal study of coronary heart disease. *Circulation,* **28,** 20.

PELL, S. & D'ALONZO, C. A. (1960). Diabetes mellitus in an employed population. *J. Am. med. Ass.* **172,** 1000.

PELL, S. & D'ALONZO, C. A. (1961). A three-year study of myocardial infarction in a large employed population. *J. Am. med. Ass.* **175,** 139.

SAILER, S., SANDHOFER, F. & BRAUNSTEINER, H. (1966). Overweight and triglyceride levels in normal persons and patients with diabetes mellitus. *Metabolism,* **15,** 135.

SPAIN, D. M. (1961). Occupational physical exertion and coronary atherosclerotic heart disease. *J. occup. Med.* **3,** 54.

STAMLER, J. (1959). The epidemiology of atherosclerotic coronary heart disease. *Post-grad. med. J.* **25,** 610, 685.

180 THE PRINCIPLES AND PRACTICE OF CLINICAL TRIALS

STAMLER, J., LINDBERG, H. A., BERKSON, D. M., SHAFFER, A., MILLER, W. & POINDEXTER, A. (1960). Prevalence and incidence of coronary heart disease in strata of the labor force of a Chicago industrial corporation. *J. chron. Dis.* **11**, 405.

STAMLER, J., BERKSON, D. M., LINDBERG, H. A., MILLER, W. & HALL, Y. (1961). Racial patterns of coronary heart disease. Blood pressure, body weight and serum cholesterol in Whites and Negroes. *Geriatrics,* **16**, 382.

STONE, M. C. & THORP, J. M. (1966). A new technique for the investigation of the low density lipoproteins in health and disease. *Clinica chim. Acta,* **14**, 812.

SYMPOSIUM (1957). Measuring the risk of coronary heart disease in adult population groups. *Am. J. publ. Hlth,* **47**, 4, Part 2.

SYMPOSIUM (1960). Prevention and control of heart disease. *Am. J. publ. Hlth,* **50**, 3, Part 2.

THOMAS, C. B. (1958). Familial and epidemiological aspects of coronary disease and hypertension. *J. chron. Dis.* **7**, 198.

ZUKEL, W. J., LEWIS, R. H., ENTERLINE, P. E., PAINTER, R. C., RALSTON, L. S., FAWCETT, R. M., MEREDITH, A. P. & PETERSON, B. (1959). A short-term community of the epidemiology of coronary heart disease. *Am. J. publ. Hlth,* **49**, 1630.

EVALUATION OF CHEMOTHERAPEUTIC DRUGS IN LEUKAEMIA AND THE RETICULOSES

J. S. MALPAS

The evaluation of chemotherapeutic agents will be discussed in general terms and an attempt made to provide some guide for the assessment of these drugs. Examples will be taken mainly from the field of leukaemia and reticular neoplasms because this is an area where progress has been most rapid and chemotherapy has achieved its widest use.

There are aspects of the use of chemotherapy which may not be met with in other fields of clinical pharmacology, at least not to such a degree. The first is, of course, the emotional factors that affect the patient, his relatives, his personal physician, the clinical investigator, the pharmaceutical company involved in providing the drug, and nowadays possibly the Government or the Government's scientific advisers. With the exception of the use of methotrexate which has been shown to be able to cure cases of choriocarcinoma in women (Hertz *et al.*, 1958) chemotherapy has so far not produced a cure although alleviation of symptoms and prolongation of life may be possible. The introduction of any new drug always raises the possibility of a cure and one cannot blame the parents of the child with acute leukaemia or their family physician if they are prepared to seek someone who will provide the new remedy. Almost immediately the pharmaceutical company is in difficulty. It is difficult for them to refuse the drug in such circumstances. Nevertheless, if the drug is used in isolation in several parts of the country there may be delay in finding out about its efficacy, and without adequate documentation the recognition of serious side effects may be delayed. The clinical investigator will endorse the limitation to a few centres especially if the drug is in short supply. Finally, in these days of international competition when a better informed public is enabled to follow the international medical scene, there may be considerable pressure from a Health Ministry for information about a particular drug.

A second difficulty with the evaluation of chemotherapeutic drugs may not be apparent, for although leukaemia, for example, is a disease of fatal outcome and involves great problems in its management, it is fortunately uncommon. The annual mortality from acute lymphoblastic leukaemia in young people up to the age of 29 was, in the period 1955 to 1959 in England and Wales, 126 per million (Court Brown and Doll, 1961). It is quite evident that the number of cases that occur near to major medical centres will be small and this has rendered it difficult to answer questions about the efficacy of drugs or combinations of drugs. The Medical Research Council has under-taken a number of cooperative trials in which several centres have participated. These trials are of a very high standard but have the disadvantage that they have taken several years to complete. Inter-national organisations now exist for cooperative chemotherapy trials, and it seems inevitable that cooperation with these groups will have to be started unless chemotherapists in this country are going to be content with conducting confirmatory studies.

To turn from general observations to the study of a specific agent. It will presumably have been shown to be active against certain tumour cell lines and its toxicity assessed in a variety of animal experiments. How can its beneficial effect be measured in man?

The first problem is to record the effect of the drug. This will naturally vary with the disease being studied. The reticuloses present more of a problem in this respect than other diseases because of the great variety of symptoms and signs. Karnofsky (1968) has recom-mended the individual patient placard which is filled in and applied at 2-month intervals to a calendar chart as shown in Figure 1. This pictorial representation has the advantage of clarity and comprehen-siveness. It enables a category of response to be derived quite quickly. Although many different types of grading can be used Karnofsky's method does allow a distinction between antilymphoma effects and practical benefit to be made. When some practical benefit occurs without evidence of any measurable antilymphoma activity it is often difficult to record.

CATEGORIES OF RESPONSE

Category 0. No clinically useful effect on the course of the disease.

   0 - 0   Disease progresses—no objective or subjective benefit.

   0 - A   Subjective benefit without favourable objective changes.

   0 - B   Favourable objective changes without subjective benefit.

   0 - C   Subjective benefit and favourable objective changes in measurable criteria but of less than one month's dura-tion then the disease progresses.

Category I. Clinical benefit with favourable objective changes in all measurable criteria of the disease.

   I - A   Distinct subjective benefit with favourable objective changes in all measurable criteria for one month or more.

   I - B   Objective regression of all palpable or measurable neoplastic disease for one month or more. Reduction of more than 50 per cent in a tumour mass.

   I - C   Complete relief of symptoms and regression of all mani-festation of disease for one year or more.

Category II. Interruption or slowing in the progression of the disease without definite evidence of subjective or objective improvement.

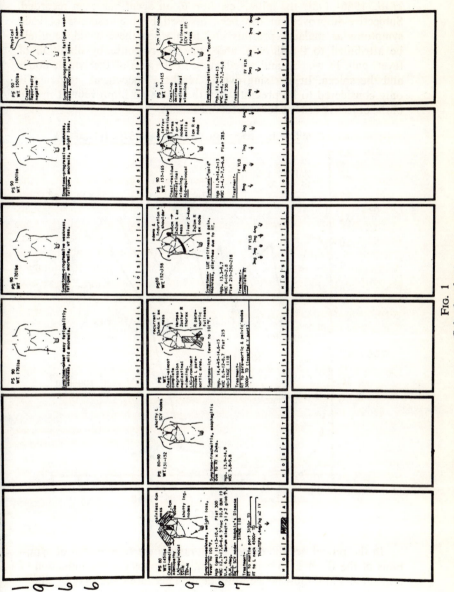

FIG. 1
Calendar chart.

In our department we have employed a rather simpler scheme assessing both objective and subjective response (Hamilton Fairley *et al.,* 1966). Only the initial response to an agent has been recorded. Subjective improvement has been assessed by the response of such symptoms as malaise, pruritus and pain when these could definitely be attributed to the disease, and objective response by abolition of fever, gain in weight, and a reduction in the size of the lymph nodes and the spleen. In assessing overall results a ' beneficial ' response is only considered to be present when there was an improvement in one of the objective criteria for at least one month.

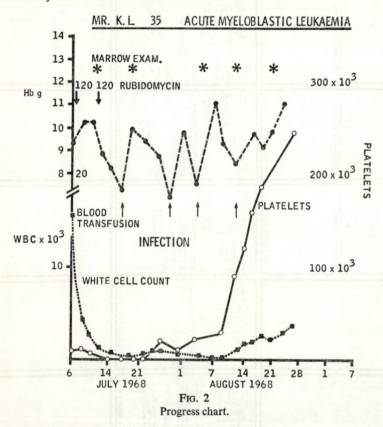

Fig. 2
Progress chart.

In the reticuloses the object of therapy is the suppression of symptoms of the disease. In acute leukaemia the object is the induction of remission, and it must be carefully defined because there may be differences between centres as to the meaning of full remission. As used in this country it means a full return of the patient to health with no clinical evidence of disease and no detectable evidence of leukaemia in the peripheral blood film. Less than 5 per cent of the cells in the

bone marrow smear should be blasts. It does not of course imply a
' cure '. The course of induction of remission and the subsequent
haematological changes is best studied by the construction of charts,
and an example of such a chart is shown in Figure 2. This illustrates
the considerable lapse of time that may occur between the administration of the agent, in this case rubidomycin, and the clinical evidence
of remission (Malpas and Bodley Scott, 1968). The method of docu-
menting the effects produced by these drugs has been dealt with at
some length, but it is essential if any satisfactory conclusions are to
be drawn.

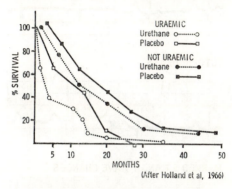

(After Holland et al, 1966)

FIG. 3
Survival in myeloma with and without
renal failure treated with urethane or a
placebo.

To return to the criteria for success. A drug producing subjective
and objective improvement may be considered successful, and one that
produces an increase in survival with a worthwhile existence will
certainly be thought so. It should not be assumed that improvement
necessarily correlates with increased survival. The use of urethane
may be taken as an example. Urethane was for more than 20 years
considered an effective and useful drug in the treatment of multiple
myeloma. It could produce both objective and subjective improvement.
Holland and his colleagues (1966) compared the effect of urethane
with a placebo in multiple myeloma. The survival of uraemic and
non-uraemic patients treated with urethane or the placebo is shown
in Figure 3. The worst survival rates are seen in those patients with
renal failure. In both groups, however, the patients treated with the
placebo do somewhat better. The worst survival rates are seen in
uraemic patients treated with urethane. The probable explanation is
that urethane induced nausea, vomiting and dehydration, and precipi-
tated deterioration into acute renal failure.

In acute leukaemia, because of the relatively short survival in the
untreated patient, one of the most satisfactory and secure measure-

ments is prolongation of survival, and in particular the measurement of median survival. Because the length of survival has been shown to depend on whether the patient goes into remission, the rate of induction of remission can also be used as a guide to the efficacy of a drug. It must be emphasised that in assessing the claims of any centre their criteria for remission must be studied with care.

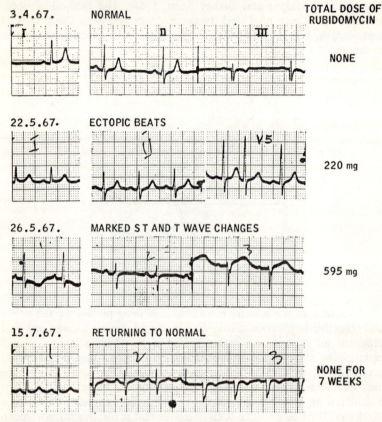

FIG. 4
Electrocardiographic changes in rubidomycin therapy.

Having decided what to measure, the next step is how the drug can be introduced for clinical trial. In deciding this a most important consideration may be the natural history of the disease, and the success, or otherwise, of agents already employed. It is difficult, for instance, to introduce new agents into the therapy of acute lymphoblastic leukaemia in children, certainly as far as a full formal trial is concerned, because the combination of prednisolone and vincristine already produce remission rates of the order of 80 to 90 per cent. On the other hand, the disastrous course of adult acute myeloblastic leukaemia and the relative ineffectiveness of the drugs so far introduced make it quite ethical to use any drug which in preliminary studies has been shown to have an effect. 'Preliminary studies' has been used advisedly because as so frequently stressed in this symposium there must be two stages to the introduction of any drug. The initial stage must be its use in a variety of malignancies at different dosage and by different routes of administration. As an example of how important the route of administration may be, methotrexate has been shown to be far more effective in maintaining remission when given intermittently by parenteral administration compared with continuous oral dosage (Selawry and Frei, 1964). It is therefore important not to put a new drug into an elaborate trial immediately. Unknown aspects of its toxicity may prevent its use as prescribed in the protocol. This will result in cooperative groups being unable to give it, they may become disillusioned and chaos will result. An example of how an intensive study in a small number of patients in a pilot trial sometimes helps to define a toxic effect and provide a method for its early detection is our experience with rubidomycin. We were able to demonstrate that the electrocardiogram will show severe cardiotoxicity, and that the cardiotoxic effect is dose dependent (Fig. 4). In our first 12 patients treated there were two cases of cardiotoxicity, one of whom died. With careful monitoring there was no further serious toxicity in 20 cases.

It is also true that one may be full of foreboding over a particular feature which is later found not to be important: 'If hopes were dupes, fears may be liars' (A. H. Clough: *Say Not the Struggle Naught Availeth*). In the Medical Research Council trial of treatment of acute leukaemia in adults (1966), where a comparison of steroid and mercaptopurine therapy alone and in combination was made, some physicians held it to be wrong that 6-mercaptopurine should be used in the presence of a low platelet count. They felt that 6-mercaptopurine would lower the platelet count still further and the patients would die from haemorrhage. When the

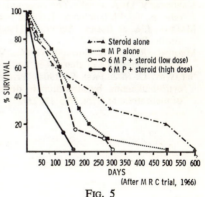

Survival in acute lymphoblastic leukaemia in adults treated by four methods.

survival in the various groups was assessed (Fig. 5) it can be seen that 6-mercaptopurine had little serious effect; it was, in fact, the group treated by high dosage of steroids that did badly.

When the drug has passed preliminary studies and been shown to be effective, it must then be considered for a formal trial and should probably be compared with the best types of therapy previously available. It must be used in such a way that an answer will be obtained. We have already had in this symposium the pitfalls in designing clinical trials pointed out very clearly, but there is always the temptation, sometimes irresistible, to try to answer too many questions at once. With regard to chemotherapy the aims of the trial should be clearly defined, one, or at the most two, problems posed, the cooperative centres should be large enough and have sufficient number of patients to obtain an answer within about a year, the centres must have facilities to be able to manage problems produced as side effects of the drugs used, platelet transfusion in thrombocytopenia, for example, and statistical advice must be available to say when the trial should be stopped.

REFERENCES

COURT BROWN, W. M. & DOLL, R. (1961). Leukaemia in childhood and young adult life. *Br. med. J.* **1**, 981.

HAMILTON FAIRLEY, G., PATTERSON, M. J. L. & BODLEY SCOTT, R. (1966). Chemotherapy of Hodgkin's disease with cyclophosphamide, vinblastine and procarbazine. *Br. med. J.* **2**, 75.

HERTZ, R., BERGENSTAL, D. M., LIPSETT, M. B., PRICE, E. B. & HILBISH, T. F. (1958). Chemotherapy of choriocarcinoma and related trophoblastic tumours in women. *J. Am. med. Ass.* **168**, 845.

HOLLAND, J. F., HOSELEY, H., SCHARLAU, C., CARBONE, P. P., FREI, E., BRINDLEY, C. O., HALL, T. C., SHNIDER, B. I., GOLD, G. L., LASAGNA, L., OWENS, A. H. & MILLER, S. P. (1966). A controlled trial of urethane treatment in multiple myeloma. *Blood*, **27**, 328.

KARNOFSKY, D. A. (1968). *The International Conference on Leukaemia-Lymphoma*, p. 409. Philadelphia : Lea and Febiger.

MALPAS, J. S. & BODLEY SCOTT, R. (1968). Rubidomycin in acute leukaemia in adults. *Br. med. J.* **3**, 227.

MEDICAL RESEARCH COUNCIL (1966). Working party on the evaluation of different methods of therapy in leukaemia. *Br. med. J.* **1**, 1383.

SELAWRY, O. S. & FREI, S. (1964). Prolongation of remission in acute lymphocytic leukaemia by alteration in dose schedule and route of administration of methotrexate. *Clin. Res.* **12**, 231.

EVALUATION OF PSYCHOTROPIC DRUGS

(1) IN SCHIZOPHRENIA

G. R. DANIEL

The principles on which psychotropic drugs are tested in humans are similar to those for other drugs. That is to say, they include initial testing in human volunteers, followed by basic studies on patients. At an early stage particular attention is paid to absorption and distribution and to toxicity. After an attempt has been made to obtain some sort of a dose response curve, many controlled trials are carried out, and unwanted reactions and interactions with other drugs are recorded. At the same time, lengthy studies of long-term clinical and toxic effects are made.

The purpose of this paper is to review the methods for assessing one group of psychotropic drugs, the major tranquillisers. These include such groups of drugs as the phenothiazines and butyrophenones. Although they are used for several psychiatric conditions, it is their assessment in controlling the schizophrenic with which this paper is concerned.

As the major tranquillisers exert little pharmacological effect on normal subjects, the main value of these earliest studies lies in the assessment of their toxicity and unwanted reactions. At some time during its early evaluation, specific toxicity tests such as the effect of the drug on the electrocardiogram and electroencephalogram should be carried out as well as normal laboratory and physiological procedures. Special attention should also be paid to its effect on liver function, pulse and blood pressure.

Because of the lack of suitable animal models and because studies in normal volunteers yield little information which suggests its eventual clinical utility, the drug is tested on patients with a wide variety of psychiatric and, perhaps, other illnesses. Let us suppose, however, that it is likely to have a tranquillising action in schizophrenia. If the early studies are performed by clinicians with a wide experience in the assessment of drugs in this condition, there is no need for control groups. Such measures restrict dose manipulation and the free evaluation of the drug. An uncontrolled study can usually answer more questions than the controlled trial and the investigator is better able to get a feel of the drug's potentialities. Any hunches may later be proved or disproved by conventional double-blind procedures. It is with these controlled trials that this paper is principally concerned and, since it is the investigator's aim to design a trial where variables are eliminated or controlled, the subject is reviewed with this in mind.

When the earliest studies have demonstrated clinical utility within a certain dose range, several kinds of controlled trials are devised. Each will explore certain features of the drug: the nature of its activity, possibly its value in special sub-groups of schizophrenia, its speed of action, its long-term clinical activity and its short- and long-term toxicity. The ideals which are arrived at are presented here but it is inevitable that in practice certain compromises will be made.

Trials in acutely psychotic patients provide the best data because of the dramatic response which an effective drug can produce. In many trials carried out by the National Institute of Mental Health in the U.S.A. only those patients admitted in an acute state are included in the trial. In every instance the criteria for the selection of patients must be agreed by all investigators during the planning stage. These criteria will be discussed later in some detail for it is in this area that some of the most important variables exist. For the purposes of the trial, no patient should have received an *effective* dose of a major tranquilliser for at least a week, and preferably a month, before admission. Ideally the patient should have received no tranquilliser at all for that month, but relapsing schizophrenics—which account for about 70 per cent of the hospital admissions for schizophrenia—have usually received some medication during that month. If they are admitted late in the afternoon or overnight, and appear to be possible candidates for the trial, they can be given barbiturates before the investigators assess them. Because of observer errors and observer differences, it is desirable that two investigators assess each patient throughout the trial. Unfortunately, because of lack of staff, holidays, and other factors, this is not often possible. After the first assessment the patients are given the standard or test drug according to a random code unknown to the patient and all those involved in the patient's assessment. Methods for measuring response to the drug will be considered in detail later. A standard starting dose for each drug is agreed upon before the trial and this can be altered in a blind fashion by increasing or decreasing the dose by fixed amounts and (if speed of action is to be compared) at fixed intervals. This dosage method is a little inflexible and presupposes that equipotent doses for the standard and test drugs are already known. If dosage has to be changed many times during the first two or three weeks, then relative speed of action cannot be properly assessed. Another way of altering doses is to have a psychiatrist not associated with the trial look either at the patient or the rating cards and prescribe in a non-blind fashion. However, it is likely he will know how to handle the control better than the test drug because of his previous experience with it.

If the patient does not respond adequately within a given time after the drug dosage has been raised to an agreed maximum, he should be withdrawn from the trial. Some investigators then give the patient the other drug, and for those patients the trial becomes a cross-over design. Each patient should be studied for two to three months but, after that, little further effect can be expected from the drug. Although the patients respond markedly during the first few weeks, a drug's full effect will not be noted until the patient has received it for at least three months. The longer the trial continues, however, the greater the risk of variations in the environment. For instance, the ward staff may change, patients will come and go, the ward may be decorated, amenities may alter, and the weather may change.

Many patients require medication other than those under trial during the test period. These may include hypnotics, anti-depressants, laxatives and other drugs for intercurrent illnesses. The nature and dose of such drugs as hypnotics and anti-depressants can be agreed upon before the trial. In principle, it is best to prescribe no drug other than the test and standard compounds, but this is not always ethically feasible. However, they should be given only to those who require them and assessments of depression, sleep disturbance or whatever should be made with due regard to the additional drugs used. If possible no second drug which is likely to interact or influence the absorption and fate of those under trial should be used. In practice this is not easy to achieve when little is known about the new drug.

The maintenance of the double-blind state is an important consideration. When some aspect of a patient's response suggests to the investigator which of the drugs he is receiving, the investigator may be influenced, even subconsciously, in the assessment of that patient. Often that suggestion may be wrong but the influence still exists. As long as the medications used during the trial are identical in as many respects as possible, the double-blind state will fail only if the organisation of the trial breaks down or the patient exhibits obvious clinical or side effects which are common to one drug only. Side effects usually present the greatest problem in this regard. For instance, extrapyramidal reactions are seen with most major tranquillisers; though they are far less common with chlorpromazine than with piperazine derivatives of phenothiazines such as trifluoperazine, or with butyrophenones such as haloperidol. If a subject develops extrapyramidal symptoms in a trial, in which chlorpromazine is compared with, say, trifluoperazine, the investigator will guess—probably quite rightly—that the patient is receiving trifluoperazine. To prevent this happening, either all patients on trifluoperazine or all patients on both compounds can be given an antiParkinsonian drug. Some suggest this should not be given to the chlorpromazine group since to give such a drug is not normal practice. Others suggest it is necessary because the effect of these drugs on the central nervous system may be such as to influence the patient's psychotic state. It is known, for instance, that the anti-Parkinsonian agent benzhexol can produce a psychotic state on its own.

Recently there have been several trials on fluphenazine enanthate and fluphenazine decanoate. These long-acting esters are given by intramuscular injection and control the symptoms of schizophrenia for several weeks. When they are compared with tablets the two groups of patients receive either active injection and placebo tablets or placebo injections and active tablets. The extrapyramidal reactions produced by the ester are most obvious during the week after the injection is given, but in a trial in which oral fluphenazine was the control drug, the investigators were unable to guess the identity of the drugs with any degree of reliability, even though antiParkinsonian drugs were given only when necessary.

In a trial where chlorpromazine was compared with fluphenazine, the double-blind state broke down one day in April when the sun began to shine. Many of the patients were allowed to sit out in the open and several became sunburnt. Since chlorpromazine causes photosensitivity while fluphenazine does not, it was easy for the investigator to identify many of those on chlorpromazine.

Schizophrenics are notoriously unreliable when it comes to taking tablets. In an out-patient study, Parkes and his colleagues (1962) found that nearly one-half defaulted, while Hare and Willcox (1967) showed that approximately one in five in-patients were similarly unreliable. If possible the trial drugs should be given in the form of a syrup since some patients even spit out or regurgitate their tablets. In practice this is not easy as it is more difficult to make syrups with identical flavours and appearance. The administration of the drugs should be recorded and spot urine checks made to see if they have been absorbed.

Only a passing reference was made to the selection of patients for the trial. First of all, therefore, let us consider the diagnosis of schizophrenia. Essentially this must be clearly defined and agreed upon by all investigators; for what is meant by schizophrenia to one psychiatrist may be significantly different to another. Psychiatrists with radical ideas have little to offer in the assessment of drugs for their results can be of personal or local interest only. Every endeavour should be made, therefore, to have investigators with equal experience and similar and representative ideas about the condition. If they all come from the same school so much the better. Ideally they should also have similar personality traits so that there is some similarity in the doctor-patient relationship. Agreement on diagnosis is an important consideration. It is worth recalling that there are many studies demonstrating observer variations in the assessment of electrocardiograms, clinical signs in the chest and even in the blood pressure. Small wonder, therefore, that there are poor correlations in the assessment of psychiatric conditions where diagnoses are based on subjective impressions. For instance, in a study by Rawnsley (1966) 30 case summaries were given to psychiatrists in England and Wales and there was a substantial measure of agreement on diagnosis. However, when these were submitted to psychiatrists in Denmark, Norway, Sweden and the U.S.A. there was wide disagreement. Where the Europeans diagnosed depression, obsessional disorder or paranoid psychosis, the Americans tended to make a diagnosis of schizophrenia. There was a reasonable degree of agreement for just over two-thirds of the patients when broad diagnostic categories were employed, but at the level of sub-categories of diagnosis, it was concluded that the international differences in usage of terms was too great to make any comparisons between countries worthwhile. In another study where a group of 6,000 patients was assessed in an observation unit and later in a mental hospital, Norris (1959) found an 89 per cent agreement on category diagnosis for functional psychosis, but for that of schizophrenia only 68 per cent. It is, therefore, reasonable to suppose that many patients used in drug trials on schizophrenia are not schizophrenics. Thus, all those involved in assessing the patients' responses should discuss their criteria for diagnosis in some detail, clearly define all nomenclature used and reach agreement on the representative significance of various phenomena. In a recent trial by the National Institute of Mental Health (1967) the following criteria for the selection of patients were used:

They should be:

1. Newly admitted schizophrenics.

2. Aged between 16 and 50.

There should be:

3. Absence of unequivocal evidence of chronic or acute brain syndrome, epilepsy, mental deficiency, drug addiction, chronic alcoholism and liver damage.

4. Presence during the preceding month of at least one of the following seven target symptoms: thinking disturbance, catatonic motor behaviour, paranoid ideation; hallucinations; delusional thinking; disturbed affect (in particular blunting or inappropriateness); and disturbance of social behaviour and interpersonal relations.

The range in diagnosis must be clearly defined and limited as far as is possible so that the patient population consists of a relatively homogeneous group of schizophrenics. Not only the diagnosis but the limits of the severity of the illness should be agreed upon. Many rating scales consist of target symptoms against which scores are set. These scores may be added up and used as a measurement of the severity of the illness. Certain limits in the scores can then be set on the trial population. The response of a psychiatric patient may be influenced considerably by the background and circumstances in which the examination is carried out. The setting for the patient's examination should not vary and should be standardised for all those in the trial. To lessen observer errors it is advisable that two investigators assess the patients at every phase of the trial. Some consider that assessments can be made at one interview by both, while others believe that such an arrangement is unsatisfactory for the patient. If interviews are made independently, it is necessary that there should be as short a gap as possible between the assessments to avoid fluctuations in the patient's clinical state. This is not as important as in the case of depressed patients, however, where there can be a marked diurnal variation in mood.

Having considered the diagnosis and the definition of the patient population, let us now look at the methods used for assessing their response to drugs. First it must be realised that any change in a patient's condition is not due to the drug only but to a large number of factors, all of which are interrelated. For instance, a relapsing schizophrenic is readmitted to hospital usually because of an increase in environmental stress and because he has stopped taking his tranquillisers. The mere effect of hospitalisation may produce a significant improvement since he has been removed from the stressful situation outside. His attitude towards the doctors, nurses and fellow patients —and their attitude towards him—may markedly influence the course of the illness. His attitude towards hospitalisation is important, his motivation to get well, his personality and his habits—all are variables which influence the patient's response. To an extent these can be measured by psychological tests but it is difficult to divorce the drug's effect from these variables, not only because all are not measurable but because each factor is influenced by the others. Lastly, and more important, any psychotherapy or occupational therapy given is likely to produce a positive response which will not be uniform for all patients.

Measurements of physiological function and biochemical tests are of little value in the assessment of drug effects so that virtually all are of a subjective nature. The check list of symptoms and questionnaires have been developed into the so-called rating scale, and this is used to record the opinion of the investigator in a systematic fashion. It should be so constructed as to encompass all those symptoms and phenomena likely to occur in the defined patient population during the trial period. If the patients cannot be assessed adequately on such a scale, then the scale is wrong. As mentioned before, each of the target symptoms should be defined at the start of the trial. Further, the degrees of severity should be graded and understood by all the investigators, and not just labelled as ' nil ', ' moderate ' or ' marked ', or on a numbered scale. Since the composition of a good rating scale is a difficult procedure, a would-be investigator should study those available and choose one best suited to his own ideas, the patient population and the circumstances of the trial. He should then test and re-test it on the same patient to assess his own reliability and the scale's sensitivity. Next, he should compare his ratings with those of his co-investigators to assess the degree of correlation and discuss in detail any disagreements in ratings between them. Lastly, he should be sufficiently experienced with the scale that its use is not just experimental for the first few patients.

Some rating scales have numerical scores for each of the symptoms and these are sometimes weighted so that when all are added up a fair assessment of the patient's overall clinical state is given. Others have a space for a general assessment. In the National Institute of Mental Health studies, two general assessment scales have been used —one to rate the severity of the illness on a seven-point scale from ' normal—no illness ' to ' amongst the most severely ill ', and another to assess the degree of improvement on a seven-point scale ranging from ' very much improved ' to ' very much worse '.

In Great Britain psychological tests are infrequently used in clinical trials, though the behavioural aspects of the condition deserve some assessment. While the rating of symptomatology is made by the psychiatrist, that of ward behaviour is usually made by nurses who have the patients under close observation for prolonged periods. In my experience these have been of limited value because of the un-reliable rating by the nurses involved. Ideally all nurses should practise using the behaviour scale before the trial starts; they should also assess their reliability by rating the same patients twice and, where more than one nurse is involved, obtain a high degree of correlation between one and another. Occasionally, their enthusiasm for the trial or lack of it can affect the patient's condition and his response to questions. Similarly, the nurse's enthusiasm or lack of it may affect the assess-ments he or she makes.

As a matter of routine, patients should always be rated by the same person and the number of ratings kept to a minimum. Only when it is necessary to assess the speed of action of the drug, or to make frequent adjustments to the dose, should multiple assessments be made. As with trials on other drugs, each rating should be made on a separate sheet of paper so that the rater cannot be influenced by the previous scores.

Over the past 10 years a plethora of rating scales, both for symptoms and behaviour, have been developed. This number indicates the problems and disagreement which abound in the assessment of the psychiatric patient. It would be impossible to discuss sufficient of them in detail and it is suggested that any involved in such trials should choose one of the scales listed in the light of preceding comments.

In addition to the use of symptom and behaviour scales, measure-ments of drug response have been made by assessing the patient's work capacity. For instance, if a patient has carried out repetitive work such as the filling of cartons with tubes in an industrial workshop, the number filled in a given time can reflect the patient's state at that time. Such scales are of use, not so much at the time of an acute relapse, but during a period of rehabilitation.

It would be wrong not to mention the evaluation of drugs in long-stay in-patient schizophrenics. Recently these have come in for a great deal of criticism and often quite justifiably so. For instance, the chronic effects of the condition and of institutionalisation may cloud the patient's psychotic symptomatology if, indeed, it still exists. However, most hospitals still have a nucleus of chronic actively-psychotic patients who can be used as a ready source of supply for drug trials. Imlah has a group of such in-patients and has used them in a number of useful clinical studies. In other centres, groups of chronic in-patients are given a placebo and if and when they relapse (this may take anything from a few days to a year or more) they may be given the test or standard drug for a fixed period. If a cross-over design is used, then the patients should be allowed to relapse before the second test period. This method demands great enthusiasm and dedication from the nursing staff and a careful assessment of the degree of relapse to which the patients should be allowed to go.

The number of patients included in most trials is less than 100 and frequently not more than 50. Unless it is the investigator's purpose to assess differential drug responses in various sub-types of schizophrenia, there is little to be gained by using large numbers. Some studies have attempted to use scales which measure the effects of drugs on certain sub-types of schizophrenia. Goldberg's analysis (1968) of a study of the National Institutes of Health is an example of this. Hamilton (1960) has also written extensively on the use of factor analysis in psychiatric drugs trials. If statistically significant differences cannot be shown with small numbers then it may be that there is no difference of clinical importance. Since the statistical evaluation of psychiatric trials is more complex than most it is advisable to employ the services of a good medical statistician, otherwise a faulty trial design may be used or incorrect statistical methods applied to useful data.

Obviously the suggestions given in this chapter indicate how trials could be carried out given the ideal conditions. In practice, there usually has to be a compromise. With the lack of large research centres and, of course, large homogeneous groups of patients, the ideal trial is a Utopian dream. Multicentre trials are best carried out by bodies such as the National Institutes of Mental Health in the United States, or the Medical Research Council and the Royal Medico-Psychological Association in Great Britain. These trials, unfortunately, introduce large numbers of variables which can be difficult to control and nobody lightly embarks on such ventures.

Few trials have shown obvious statistical differences between any of the phenothiazines and this is probably because of variable factors, and because the assessment of response is relatively inaccurate. However, these must not act as an absolute deterrent to carrying out such studies or no new drugs would be tested.

REFERENCES

Tablet defaulting

HARE, E. H. & WILLCOX, D. R. C. (1967). Do psychiatric in-patients take their pills? *Br. J. Psychiat.* **113**, 1435.

PARKES, C. M., BROWN, G. W. & MONCK, E. M. (1962). The general practitioner and the schizophrenic patient. *Br. med. J.* **1**, 972.

Diagnostic reviews

NORRIS, V. (1959). *Mental Illness in London,* Maudsley Monograph No. 6. London: Chapman and Hall.

RAWNSLEY, K. (1966). *Fourth World Congress of Psychiatry,* Madrid. (Not in Published Proceedings.)

National Institute of Mental Health Studies

GOLDBERG, S. C. & MATTSSON, N. B. (1968). Schizophrenic subtypes defined by response to drugs and placebo. *Dis. nerv. Syst.* **29**, No. 5 (Suppl.), 153.

NATIONAL INSTITUTE OF MENTAL HEALTH, Psychopharmacology Service Center Collaborative Study Group (1964). Phenothiazine treatment in acute schizophrenia. *Archs gen. Psychiat.* **10**, 246.

NATIONAL INSTITUTE OF MENTAL HEALTH, Psychopharmacology Research Branch Collaborative Study Group (1967). Differences in clinical effects of three phenothiazines in ' acute ' schizophrenia. *Dis. nerv. Syst.* **28**, 369.

Rating scales

BAKER, A. A. & THORPE, J. G. (1956). Some simple measures of schizophrenic deterioration. *J. ment. Sci.* **102**, 838.
Ward Behaviour Scale.

BURDOCK, E. I., HAKEREM, G., HARDESTY ANNES, & ZUBIN, J. (1960). A Ward Behaviour Rating Scale for mental patients. *J. clin. Psychol.* **16**, 246.

HAMILTON, M., SMITH, A. L. G., LAPIDUS, H. E. & CADOGAN, E. P. (1960). A controlled trial of thiopropazate dihydrochloride (Dartalan), chlorpromazine and occupational therapy in chronic schizophrenics. *J. ment. Sci.* **106**, 40.
A modification of Lorr's Scale for psychiatrists and nurses.

LORR, M., KLETT, C. J., MCNAIR, D. M. & LASKY, J. J. (1963). *In-patient Multidimensional Psychiatric Scale* (Manual). Palo Alto: Consulting Psychologists Press.

MALAMUD, W. & SANDS, S. L. (1947). A revision of the psychiatric rating scale. *Am. J. Psychiat.* **104**, 231.

OVERALL, J. E. & GORHAM, D. R. (1962). The brief psychiatric rating scale. *Psychol. Rep.* **10**, 799.

WING, J. K. (1961). A simple and reliable subclassification of chronic schizophrenia. *J. ment. Sci.* **107**, 862.
Psychiatric Rating, and Ward Behaviour Scale.

WING, J. K., BIRLEY, J. L. T., COOPER, J. E., GRAHAM, P. & ISAACS, A. D. (1967). Reliability of a procedure for measuring and classifying ' present psychiatric state '. *Br. J. Psychiat.* **113**, 499.
Being used for a W.H.O. Study on schizophrenia.

RECOMMENDED READING

Books

INTERNATIONAL ENCYCLOPAEDIA OF PHARMACOLOGY AND THERAPEUTICS (1966). Section 6, *Clinical Pharmacology,* Vol. 1, Chap. 10 and 11. Oxford: Pergamon.

14

JOYCE, C. R. B. (1968). *Psychopharmacology. Dimensions and Perspectives.* London: Tavistock.

SHEPHERD, M. (1968). *Clinical Psychopharmacology.* London: English Universities Press.

Papers

KREITMAN, N. (1961). The reliability of psychiatric diagnosis. *J. ment. Sci.* **107**, 876.

KREITMAN, N. (1961). The reliability of psychiatric assessment: an analysis. *J. ment. Sci.* **107**, 887.

EVALUATION OF PSYCHOTROPIC DRUGS

(2) DEPRESSION

PART I — 1959

M. SHEPHERD

Quantitative methods play a major part in the evaluation of new therapeutic substances. Much of the pioneer work in this field dates from 1931 when the Medical Research Council of Great Britain set up its Therapeutic Trials Committee which soon established the medical statistician as a member of the team alongside the clinician and pharmacologist (Green, 1954). In the clinical assessment of a new drug it is now generally agreed that after the basic pharmacological data have been acquired from preliminary animal experiments and from pilot trials on human subjects the information should be applied to the measurement of specified reactions against different doses of the drug. It is also necessary to establish the relationship of these reactions to the outcome of the disorder, a step which entails some knowledge of the course of the condition either without treatment or with some other form of treatment. It is then possible to proceed to the organisation of the therapeutic trial which, in its classical form, is designed to compare the effects of treatment in two or more groups to each of which there has been random allocation of patients differing only in respect of the treatment administered. The criteria of response to treatment should be as unambiguous as possible and a member of the Statistical Research Unit of the M.R.C. has pointed out that '. . . whenever possible objective and preferably measured assessment of the progress of patients should be used. It is, however, probable that this will have to be supplemented by subjective assessment' (Sutherland, 1958). Unfortunately the difficulty of standardising subjective responses has led to their virtual neglect in this field until recent years.

The controlled therapeutic trial is not, of course, necessary for the assessment of all remedies. Such trials can be dispensed with if a previously fatal condition is treated successfully—as in the case of the treatment of tuberculous meningitis by streptomycin—or when the new agent is clearly superior to its predecessors—as in the case of the treatment of scrub typhus by chloramphenicol. Further, ethical considerations may limit the possibilities of a clinical trial in some instances, especially if there is evidence to suggest that irreversible harm could be prevented by the administration of an existing treatment. Nonetheless, in so far as it has introduced the well-tried principles of prophylactic evaluation into experimental therapeutics, the modern clinical trial enforces a healthy respect for scientific method in a field where it has not always been prominent. It is important to remember at the same time that the comparative trial is essentially an epidemiological procedure and reflects the outlook of the statistician, who inevitably tends to think less as a physician and more as a metaphysician, specialising therefore in the description of the types of proof which are appropriate to various types of statement. The commonest form in which these statements are made about the therapeutic value of psychotropic drugs has led to clinical trials designed to answer questions of this order: Are patients suffering from condition X more likely to benefit from treatment A than from treatment B (which may be a placebo)? Whether such a question can be answered with confidence depends in large measure on the precision with which it is possible to define the clinical condition and to specify the criteria of benefit. On both these counts depressive states raise particular problems.

The definition and scope of the illnesses to be treated is of prime importance for the construction of representative samples. No classification of affective conditions in clinical terms can yet be more than provisional, and recent work purporting to distinguish depressive syndromes by means of the mathematical analysis of symptom-clusters has largely confirmed the judgement of clinical experience. There is a wide variation in the estimated frequency of these illnesses based on the most reliable figures we possess, namely the large-scale national statistics of hospital admissions. In England and Wales the manic-depressive psychoses, most of them in the form of depressive states, make up the largest diagnostic group among cases admitted to mental hospitals. By contrast, in the United States and Scandinavian countries—where hospital statistics are also carefully compiled—the manic-depressive psychoses and involutional melancholia combine to form a relatively small proportion of cases and schizophrenia is the condition diagnosed most frequently. This discrepancy cannot be explained wholly by true differences of prevalence. Idiosyncratic classification is partly responsible: the ' psychogenic psychoses' of the Scandinavian authors, for example, include a number of illnesses which would be regarded as depressive elsewhere. In addition, the traditions of diagnostic practice itself can affect the relative estimates of the two major functional psychoses; thus American psychiatrists appear to be guided more than we in Great Britain by Nolan Lewis's dictum that '. . . the diagnosis of manic-depressive psychoses can be made only by the elimination of schizophrenia' (Lewis and Piotrowski, 1954). The various prevalence rates of depressive illness provided by responsible workers indicate the need to consider as well the degree of disability leading to inclusion in the diagnostic category. Thus Fremming's surprisingly high figures from the island of Bornholm

(1951) must be interpreted in the light of his painstaking survey methods and of the finding that 40 per cent of his cases had not been under psychiatric care. Our experience in Great Britain has shown that patients suffering from the milder forms of depressive illness have tended to enter mental hospitals in increasing numbers as provision for treatment on a voluntary basis has been extended (Walker, 1958) and that many other cases require extra-mural services for their detection.

It is apparent that if disregarded this clinical diversity will undermine the structure of a comparative trial which depends on commensurate severity of illness in the treated and control groups. But in addition the groups must be homogeneous in respect of outcome if comparison is to be valid. Here the tendency of depressive illnesses to run a self-limiting and often recurrent course renders prognosis difficult in even the better-defined syndromes. It is also necessary to take cognizance of the appreciable mortality rate which is carried by the major depressive psychoses. Norris (1959), for example, has recently shown that the crude death rates for men and women suffering from these conditions are respectively nine and six times the corresponding rates for persons of 16 years or more in the general population.

When reasonably homogeneous groups can be constructed, the indices of response have to be defined. The clinical pharmacologist who employs quantitative methods to compare therapeutic substances may proceed by employing one of three methods (Gaddum, 1954). These are the direct assay, in which measurement is made of the dose just necessary to produce an effect; the measured response of a dependent variable; and the assay by quantal, or all or none, responses which are not measured but recorded as being present or absent. With these techniques it is possible to study dose-response data according to the conditions of the experiment. Unfortunately the disturbances of function which accompany depressive states are insufficiently constant or sensitive to be employed in the way in which, for example, blood pressure can be used in the evaluation of hypotensive agents. This is true even of those physiological indices, like weight and certain autonomic responses, as well as those psychological concomitants like the altered psychomotor reactions, which are related intimately enough to some depressive illnesses to bear on prognosis. Eugen Bleuler (1910-12) commented of melancholia that 'the affect is the index of the whole picture', and most of the reported physical and psychological changes must still be regarded as epiphenomena. For this reason, in our present state of knowledge the outcome of depressive illnesses, and the response to treatment, have still to be expressed usually in the holistic terms of clinical and social morbidity.

Ethical considerations demand that patients included in a clinical trial should not be deprived of the best available therapy. In many of the milder depressive illnesses this often comprises some non-specific form of pharmacological treatment or some form of psychotherapy. For a large proportion of the more severe illnesses, however, electrical shock therapy is available and cannot be lightly withheld for the experimental testing of a new compound. In all comparisons it is necessary to bear in mind that ECT, which despite much work and speculation remains an empirical procedure, carries a negligible mortality rate and that there are relatively few physical contraindications to its application when administered correctly. It is, nevertheless, a traumatic procedure which many patients and physicians find distasteful. Convulsive therapy has not been subjected to a formal therapeutic trial; most attempts at evaluation have been based on a comparison between the outcome of illnesses treated by ECT in hospital and the outcome of illnesses recorded by hospital controls in the pre-shock era (Ødegaard, 1954). These studies have shown that convulsive treatment reduces hospital mortality rates among patients with depressive illnesses (Slater, 1951) and that it also reduces the time which many of these patients spend in hospital (Mayer-Gross, 1951).

Only 20 years ago mental hospitals could demonstrate the spectacle of whole wards containing ' . . . chronic melancholics, who had been in the hospital for two to over twenty years. They had lost the sharp edge of their depression but were anergic, almost inaccessible to stimulation and preoccupied with delusions of unworthiness, hopelessness and physical illness which gravely incapacitated them. Some spontaneously remitted, but there were always others to take their place ' (Cook, 1958). This corner of mental hospital life has mostly disappeared following the introduction of ECT. Several workers have since used the duration of stay in hospital as a useful indication of the severity of illness. They have shown that ECT can cut short and fragment many depressive reactions, particularly in the involutional period, but that it does not influence the disease-cycle of the individual patient who exhibits periodic attacks. Further, ECT is without detectable benefit in a proportion of cases from which, on clinical grounds, favourable response would be anticipated.

At the present time there is no pharmacological substance whose efficacy can match that of ECT in the treatment of major depressive illnesses. Many drugs have been tried and found wanting—amphetamine and its congeners, the barbiturates, endocrine preparations, dinitrile succinate, methylphenidate and iproniazid, to mention only a few—but it is now more necessary than ever to specify our expectations of any effective substances which may become available. Even though a drug were to be introduced on an empirical basis it would, of course, be necessary to ensure that it was without serious side effects and that it was of low toxicity. This lesson has been very recently exemplified by iproniazid. If such a substance were no more effective than ECT it would probably find favour because of the advantages attached to its mode of administration, especially if this were by the oral route. In some instances these advantages might prove decisive even if drug therapy were in some measure inferior to ECT, for example in its speed of action. To establish its superiority over electrical treatment on clinical grounds a new drug could be responsible for one or a combination of the following effects: (1) it could reduce or abolish the mortality rate associated with depressive illnesses treated with ECT; (2) it could curtail the duration of the treated illness or mitigate the social disability still further; (3) it could prevent subsequent attacks; (4) it could prove to be efficacious in cases which had failed to respond to electrical treatment.

It is important to specify which of these features is being singled out in a comparative trial with ECT. By way of example there may be cited an experiment which we conducted with a drug reputed some years ago to be of value in the treatment of depressive states in the senium. These illnesses display several clinical and biological features in common and we attempted further to secure uniformity by choosing only patients admitted to our own geriatric unit. The patients, most of whom were in the seventh decade of life and suffering from affective illnesses uncomplicated by organic features, enjoyed in general a good prognosis, with an average period of stay in hospital of three months. It had always been the practice in this unit to assess patients for a period of time in hospital before the commencement of active treatment. Advantage was taken of this interval to introduce a double-blind procedure with drug and placebo over a period of about four weeks in which ECT was withheld. During this time blood pressure and weight were recorded, bi-weekly ratings of behaviour were made by doctors and nurses, side effects were noted and different dose schedules of drug were prescribed. Each case was reviewed at the end of this initial period, when the need for further treatment was considered and ECT was administered if it was considered necessary. The relevant results of this experiment are summarised in Table I.

Though they have not been included in the Table, the dosages of drug administered were equally distributed among all groups. From these figures it is apparent, first, that most patients required ECT after the trial period on the drug; secondly, that a successful outcome was largely associated with the administation of ECT; and thirdly, that there was no significant difference between the outcome of drug-treated and placebo-treated groups whether electrical treatment was administered or not. It was therefore possible to conclude that in the treatment of depressive illnesses with these characteristics the drug was inferior to electrical treatment and no more efficacious than the placebo.

Relatively precise answers of this type are possible even with empirical remedies, and refinements of statistical method can sharpen

TABLE I

Outcome three months after admission	Patients given ECT		Patients not given ECT	
	After placebo	After drug	After placebo	After drug
Discharged well	8	11	1	1
Discharged with symptoms	10	5	5	7
Remaining in hospital	9	12	2	1
Totals	27	28	8	9

Total number of patients = 72.

such questions by, for example, indicating the degree of improvement which would be accepted as clinically worthwhile before the trial commences (Armitage, 1954). If, however, there is a rational basis for the introduction of pharmacological treatment another order of questions becomes possible within the framework of the therapeutic experiment. Thus in a recent study carried out by Pare and Sandler (1959), iproniazid was administered to a group of depressed patients with the objectives of determining not merely whether the drug was of benefit but also whether those patients who did respond could be differentiated clinically and biochemically (by estimations of urinary 5-hydroxy-indoleacetic acid) from those who did not respond and, more specifically, whether among the positive responders there was any evidence to suggest that their response was related to changes in the brain concentration of 5-hydroxy-tryptamine (5-HT) or of catecholamines. Similarly the recent pharmacological studies which have shed light on the peripheral effects of amphetamine, particularly the liberation of norepinephrine and its 5-HT-like action, have suggested experiments to determine whether these effects are reproduced in the central nervous system of depressed patients responding to this drug. The theoretical importance of such investigations is considerable since the information obtained in a therapeutic setting may be used to shed light on the mechanism of the disorder under study. This model may receive more attention with the accumulation of relevant information about the properties of substances in current use.

The drug treatment of the less severe depressive conditions is beset by problems of its own. These reactions include the large groups of loosely termed ' neurotic ', ' reactive ', or ' exogenous ' depression often admixed with the clinical manifestations of anxiety. Many of them run a chronic, fluctuating course. In such cases depression may represent a symptom as much as a syndrome and the indices of outcome which are available for the major depressive illnesses find limited application in their treatment. Only a minority of the patients require convulsive therapy. If they do attend hospital they are unlikely to require admission and it seems probable that many of them never come under psychiatric care. Recent studies of morbidity in general practice under the National Health Service in Great Britain have suggested that depressive illnesses rank high in the psychiatric case-load of the practitioner and that he treats the majority of patients himself (Watts, 1956). It also seems probable from socio-medical inquiries that other patients suffering from these conditions do not come to medical attention at all but rely rather on the advice of the chemist or on self-medication. When the disability consists of no more than feelings of discontent, distress or discomfort, even social criteria like the work-record may be too crude for purposes of assessment.

It is notoriously difficult to apply the principles of the therapeutic trial to illnesses of this sort. Treatment can be evaluated by a group trial in favourable circumstances (Davies and Shepherd, 1955) but there are many practical and theoretical obstacles. The drop-out rate is high and there is always uncertainty as to whether the patient is taking the drug or not. The diversity within diagnostic groups is considerable and impairs the possibility of generalisation from the small numbers which are usually treated. Changes in the course of the condition may be linked more with interpersonal and social factors than with the patient's drug-treatment. The criteria of response in such trials depend, moreover, wholly or partly on clinical judgements by the observer and ratings of experience or drug-preference by the patient, criteria which are inevitably subjective. Finally, the wide individual variation of response to drugs (Von Felsinger *et al.*, 1955) assumes such importance that it may be necessary to employ an experimental design which enables the information about individuals to be extracted.

An alternative method of tackling this problem is to concentrate directly on the universe of the individual patient and to study the intra-individual variation. This principle is familiar to physiologists and psychologists (Jellinek, 1939; Shapiro, 1957). Its application to therapeutics has been advocated by Hogben and Sim (1953) as a means of direct examination of the stimulus-response nexus. What Hogben calls the self-controlled, self-recorded trial is designed to study the therapeutic response in states of chronic, low-grade morbidity which are not regarded as reversible and where the end-points of therapy are defined by symptomatic relief rather than by cure. The controlled investigation of subjective data in the form of symptoms is a central feature of the experimental design. Symptoms are subdivided for the purpose into those which are usually associated with disturbances of behaviour and so become open to observation (for example, anorexia) and those in which personal experiences predominate and render the subject's testimony the principal source of data (for example, referred pain). Our experience suggests that the treatment of less severe chronic depressive states can be investigated in this way. The suitable subject is invited to complete pre-designed forms bearing on specified functions and experiences. The form can be filled in at regular intervals in normal working or domestic conditions. Internal checks are provided for subjective data, and the cooperation of an observer can be enlisted for the verification of functional disturbance. After a period of observation without treatment the effects of medication can be observed, the subject remaining in ignorance of the substance which he receives.

If the initial recordings are made in hospital, the nursing staff will enable an estimate to be made of the reliability of the subject's observations. On discharge, the subject's spouse can cooperate in the same way for regular recordings in the intervals between psychiatric assessments. Though the technique raises several problems in the selection of subjects, the recording of information and the mathematical treatment of summated indices, the data which it provides about natural fluctuations and the continuity of response make it a promising research tool in the study of these elusive conditions.

It now seems probable that we are soon to be presented with so many new anti-depressive compounds that the familiar clinical attitude of laissez-faire empiricism will be increasingly difficult to sustain. The clinician is compelled to hold the balance between the scales of laboratory data on the one hand and stochastic theory on the other. Though his experience and judgement are essential it will be necessary for him to adopt a more experimental role in the future if he is to cooperate fully with the pharmacologist and the statistician, whose techniques he should understand if full weight is to be given to observations made in the clinical setting. More clinical research is indispensable to progress in the evaluation of drugs for the treatment of depression.

ACKNOWLEDGEMENT

This paper originally appeared in the *Canadian Psychiatric Association Journal* and is reproduced with the kind permission of the Editor.

REFERENCES

ARMITAGE, P. (1954). *Q. Jl Med. N.S.* **23,** 255.

BLEULER, E. (1910-1912). Affectivity, suggestibility, paranoia. *St. Hosp. Bull., N.T. N.S.* **3-4,** 481-601.

COOKE, L. C. (1958). *J. ment. Sci.* **104,** 933.

DAVIES, D. L. & SHEPHERD, M. (1955). Reserpine in the treatment of anxious and depressed patients. *Lancet,* **2,** 117.

FREMMING, G. H. (1951). The expectation of mental infirmity in a sample of the Danish population. *Occ. Pap. Eugen,* No. 7.

GADDUM, J. H. (1954). *Proc. R. Soc. Med.* **47,** 195.

GREEN, F. H. K. (1954). The clinical evaluation of remedies. *Lancet,* **2,** 1085.

HOGBEN, L. & SIM, M. (1953). *Br. J. prev. soc. Med.* **7,** 163.

JELLINEK, E. M. (1939). *The Function of Biometric Methodology in Psychiatric Research,* p. 48. American Association for the Advancement of Science, Publication No. 9.

LEWIS, N. D. C. & PIOTROWSKI, Z. A. (1954). Clinical diagnosis of manic-depressive psychosis. In *Depression,* ed. Hoche, P. H. & Zubin, J. New York: Grune and Stratton.

MAYER-GROSS, W. (1951). *Proc. R. Soc. Med.* **44,** 961.

NORRIS, V. (1959). Mental illness in London: a statistical enquiry into admission to mental hospitals. *Maudsley Monograph No. 6.* London: Chapman and Hall.

ØDEGAARD, Ø. (1954). *Ment. Hyg. Concord,* **38,** 447.

PARE, C. M. B. & SANDLER, M. (1959). A trial of iproniazid in the treatment of depression: a clinical and biochemical study. *J. Neurol. Neurosurg. Psychiat.* **22,** 247.

SHAPIRO, M. B. (1957). Experimental method in the psychological description of the individual psychiatric patient. *Int. J. soc. Psychiat.* **3,** 89.

SLATER, E. T. O. (1951). *J. ment. Sci.* **97,** 567.

SUTHERLAND, I. (1958). *A Symposium on Clinical Trials.* Pfizer.

VON FELSINGER, J. M., LASAGNA, L. & BEECHER, H. K. (1955). *J. Am. med. Ass.* **157,** 1113.

WALKER, L. D. (1958). The pattern of post-war psychiatric practice. *Thesis (M.D.)* University of London.

WATTS, C. A. H. (1956). *Neuroses in General Practice.* Royal College of Physicians Publication No. 6. Edinburgh.

EVALUATION OF PSYCHOTROPIC DRUGS

(2) DEPRESSION

PART II — 1969

M. SHEPHERD

Part I of this survey reviewed the evaluation of pharmacotherapy in the treatment of depression with special reference to the place of clinical trials. It is now appropriate, therefore, to survey some of the more important developments of the past decade in the field. For convenience the material can be grouped into four general categories: (1) attitudes to clinical trials, (2) the early evaluation of anti-depressant medication, (3) the confirmatory evaluation of anti-depressant medication and (4) the prophylaxis of depression.

Attitudes to clinical trials

Social psychologists insist that attitudes are precursors to action. As such they warrant consideration in their own right, and it is instructive to recall the opening remarks of the discussant of my 1959 paper on the subject of controlled clinical trials: ' Such studies seem to have undergone a kind of historical waxing and waning. Thus prior to the last decade or two, one seldom heard of them. Once they entered the scene, however, it became fashionable to decry the results that were not " controlled " in this manner. But now the wheel has, as it were, turned full circle so that it is fashionable, even perhaps avant garde, to heap critical coals of fire upon such an approach ' (Sloane, 1959).

Clearly the fire has largely died out since that time. The changed attitude of the pharmaceutical industry is attested by the organisation of this meeting and the excellent set of papers which have been presented by members of the industry. Many workers in the medical profession have also come to adopt a more critical attitude to therapeutics, possibly associated with the rise of clinical pharmacology as an emerging discipline, and several psychiatrists have questioned both the claims advanced on behalf of anti-depressant drugs (Kimbell et al., 1965) and the adequacy of the methods being employed to evaluate them (Leyburn, 1967). In this context one of the most instructive reports reviewed all papers concerned with the evaluation of anti-depressant medication which had been published in 17 American, British and Canadian journals over a five-year period (Wechsler et al., 1965). The authors identified 79 separate studies of which 30 had been conducted without controls, 22 with placebo controls and 27 with active drug controls.

EVALUATION OF PSYCHOTROPIC DRUGS: DEPRESSION

A more detailed analysis of the publications made it possible to draw several conclusions of general interest. First, there was considerable variability in the reports of any one medication, and assessments of efficacy ranged from nil to 100 per cent. Secondly, the type of research design was related to reported outcome: in general, studies in which placebos were employed yielded the lowest estimates of efficacy. Thirdly, in studies where placebo was used an improvement on the drug tended to be associated with improvement on the placebo. Fourthly, the administration of electro-convulsive therapy was more effective than any form of medication. It is surely important to emphasise these findings as a background to any individual study in this area.

The early evaluation of anti-depressant medication

Reviewing research in psychopharmacology a W.H.O. Scientific Group has sub-divided the stages of clinical drug evaluation into three phases (W.H.O., 1967). Phase I concentrates on a determination of the effective dose range, adverse effects and possible toxic properties of a new drug; such work depends on experience and careful clinical observation, and is usually carried out on groups of 5 to 10 patients as a therapeutic experiment without controls. Phase II trials are concerned with the therapeutic range and effectiveness of the drugs which are studied; they may or may not be controlled and should be conducted with larger groups of the order of 10 to 30 by an investigator who is apotheosized as ' a perceptive observer, able to use imagination and follow clinical " hunches ".' Together, the first and second phases of clinical trials constitute the stage of early evaluation when it is possible to make observations which can be validated by the more strictly controlled techniques of phase III.

In the sphere of anti-depressant medication the stage of early evaluation has been most neglected. Partly this is due to the difficulties posed by the use of animal behaviour for the study of affective phenomena in man. The logic of the pharmacologist may, of course, dismiss this obstacle as chimaerical, as in the following example: ' How does one study the anti-depressive action of a sedative? Obviously, normal animals cannot be used; we must somehow set up a model depression in animals. But depression does not have the same meaning to a physiologist as it does to a psychiatrist, and I did not wish to become entangled in semantic difficulties. I asked a psychiatrist friend to describe to me the symptoms of endogenous depression in a subject who had only recently acquired the disease. It seemed to me that I was listening to a description of the action of reserpine—even to its parasympathetic effects. We decided therefore that our model depression would be the syndrome of effects elicited by reserpine or reserpine-like compounds.' (Brodie, 1965.)

However satisfying such a simplified view may be to its originators, it is not supported by the experimental or clinical facts. There is still no adequate substitute for the human subject when depression is to be investigated or treated and, unfortunately, the first administration of a new anti-depressant drug to man all too often exemplifies what has justifiably been termed a ' leap in the dark '.

It was with this problem in mind, and with an awareness of the dearth of investigations designed to tackle it, that we attempted to explore some of the practical and theoretical aspects of early evalua-tion with a new anti-depressant compound at the Institute of Psychiatry two years ago. Our objectives were to examine whether the oral administration of this drug to depressed in-patients was effective and, simultaneously, to assess the side effects of the drug and its action on haematological, hepatic, renal and cardiovascular function. Inas-much as we were concerned to try and devise a method for testing new anti-depressants on a restricted number of patients before release in large scale trials we were, in effect, combining phases I and II in a single operation.

This work has been fully reported (Blackwell and Shepherd, 1967). It demonstrated conclusively how many practical and administrative hurdles lie in the path of the would-be investigator on this track. Here I would mention only one, namely the problem of obtaining suitable patients. Thus, although we were working in a large and relatively well staffed institution with access to many patients, only 6 out of the 90 depressed subjects who met the criteria for inclusion in the study completed the trial. The reasons for the heavy loss of patients included refusal of consent by patient, relative or consultant; the existence of a complicating physical condition; rapid remission or self-discharge from hospital; worsening of illness to require electro-convulsive treat-ment; and a history of previous treatment with a similar drug. It is evident that despite the mutual interest of the pharmaceutical industry and the medical profession in promoting such research its organisation demands more facilities than are generally acknowledged. Early evaluation remains an outstanding challenge if the flood of new anti-depressant drugs is to justify itself.

The confirmatory evaluation of anti-depressant medication
    In terms of the W.H.O. schema the phase III controlled trial requires larger groups of patients ' . . . so that sensitive statistical tests can be used in evaluating the final results. Phase III trials, therefore, call for carefully conceived and executed experiments and for skilful evaluation of the results '. There are, as the report further points out, no fewer than eight possible types of experimental control which may be employed. They are: the comparison of a drug with no treatment, which can be non-blind, single-blind or double-blind; the compari-son of one drug with another drug which again can be non-blind, single-blind or double-blind; and a comparison of a drug with a

placebo, which must be either single-blind or double-blind. The number of controlled trials of anti-depressant medication has been steadily increasing over the past decade, but so far the largest and the most impressive is the multi-centred investigation organised under the aegis of the Medical Research Council (Medical Research Council, 1965). The trial was designed to compare the efficacy of four treatments—ECT, a tricyclic anti-depressant, a monoamine oxidase inhibitor and a placebo—on depressed in-patients over a period of six months. Three aspects of this study are of principal interest in the context of this symposium: the criteria for selection, the methods of evaluation and the results (Shepherd, 1967a).

The criteria for inclusion of patients centred on an operational definition of depressive illness: ' The primary manifestation and major symptom of the illness to be a persistent alteration of mood (with or without diurnal variation) which exceeds customary sadness, is evident to the examiner, and is accompanied by one or more of the following symptoms: self-depreciation with a morbid sense (or delusional ideas) of guilt; sleep disturbance; hypochondriasis; retardation of thought and action; agitated behaviour '. To ensure that the characteristics of the trial-population were as homogeneous as possible the patients also had to be aged between 40 and 69 years and to be free of serious physical disease; further, the duration of their illnesses had not to exceed 18 months before their entry into the trial, and adequate treatment during the preceding 6 months constituted a bar to inclusion. In the absence of objective pathological criteria it is imperative to adopt such methods in studies of this type, though the details must of course be dependent on the sub-group of the depressive population to be studied (Shepherd, 1967b).

Secondly, there are the methods of evaluation which were adopted. These were constructed around three separate parameters: discharge from hospital, clinical ratings and what can be termed ' controlled clinical behaviour '. While discharge from hospital may be taken to indicate clinical improvement the notion was also extended to include ' final ' discharge, signifying discharge without re-admission or the administration of out-patient ECT during the six months follow-up period. The clinical ratings were made on an overall assessment of severity and on each of fifteen specified symptoms; they were recorded on a specially designed form which was constructed for this investigation and administered on admission, weekly during the first month in hospital, just before discharge and at the end of the second, third and sixth months. The meaning of clinical behaviour, i.e. the clinical decisions of participating physicians, was analysed within the regulations laid down for the conduct of the trial: if, for example, the physician chose to continue with the prescribed, randomly allocated, tablets after the fourth week of treatment—when he was permitted to adopt an alternative—it was reasonably inferred that maintenance of the original treatment indicated satisfaction with the clinical response at that point in time.

Thirdly, the results—which may be summarised baldly as follows. Approximately one-third of the patients did well on placebo and one sixth of the patients did badly despite the treatments they received; about one sixth of the patients needed ECT following an initial course of tablets, regardless of their composition; the administration of ECT and one of the two active preparations was associated with a better response than went with placebo, but the action of ECT was more rapid; the effects of the other compound could not be distinguished from the placebo-response.

No mention of such results, however, is complete without stressing that they apply only to groups of patients, and not to individuals. All attempts to identify which factors determined individual response to treatment were unsuccessful. The great variation of response within defined groups of depressed patients is clearly of considerable interest in its own right and it has recently been subjected to close analysis from three different points of view, all of which relate to the problems of therapeutic evaluation: these viewpoints are concerned respectively with (1) the classification of depressive disorders, (2) the biological basis of depression, and (3) the social factors bearing on depression.

1. The importance of an adequate system of classification is apparent. If, as some workers maintain, there are several aetiologically distinct types of depressive illness it would not be surprising to find that our relatively crude clinical criteria fail to distinguish between heterogeneous conditions which respond differentially to the same treatment. Within the limitations of our present knowledge perhaps the most adequate solution has been proposed by Kendell (1968) on the basis of his analysis of a large series of depressive illnesses with refined statistical methods. His conclusion was '. . . to regard depressive illnesses as a continuum, with the classical neurotic depressions at one pole, the classical endogenous depression at the other and the majority of patients in between.' Further, he goes on to suggest that a mathematically derived index of the condition along the lines he has developed can be substituted usefully for clinical concepts: 'To say that a patient has a depressive illness with an index score of +4 is more informative than saying that he has a psychotic depression or even that he has a borderline psychotic depression'. Here is a line of research which can be adopted profitably in therapeutic experimentation.

2. The biological explanation of the variations in therapeutic response tends to focus on drug-metabolism and this emphasis sometimes leads to direct criticism of the clinical trial in its usual form: '. . . a biologist sounds a word of warning when he hears that " double-blind " studies are carried out using fixed dosage schedules. The double-blind test involves a sound principle and is meant to separate

factors such as variability of the disease process, bias, placebo effects, and so forth. But the use of this test implies that the drug is present in each subject in approximately the same amount in mg/kg. This might be true with highly polar drugs, substances which are not metabolised and disappear from the body at rates that are essentially similar among different individuals. In contrast, drugs that act on the brain, being highly lipid soluble, undergo extensive metabolism at rates that are highly variable from person to person. Thus, the investigator applying the double-blind test in the belief that he is circumventing biological variability, may be substituting a situation in which the biological variability is vastly greater ' (Brodie, 1965).

The study of individual differences in human drug metabolism is pre-eminently a task for the clinical pharmacologist. Technical reasons have handicapped its application to the anti-depressant field until recently, but the development of new chemical methods have now enabled some workers to demonstrate its relevance. In Stockholm, for example, a sensitive in vitro labelling technique has been used to estimate the plasma level of monomethylated tricyclic anti-depressants in man. Figure 1 illustrates the range of individual variation in the plasma levels of desmethylimipramine and also, incidentally, the interesting observation that disturbing side-effects were associated with high plasma-levels of desmethylimipramine (Sjöqvist *et al.*, 1968).

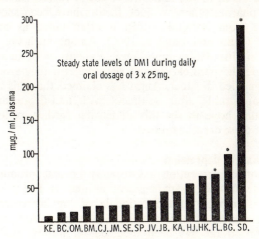

FIG. 1

Individual differences in plasma concentrations (steady-state) of desmethylimipramine. Each bar is based on 3-5 determinations S.D.<10 per cent (Modified after Hammer and Sjöqvist, 1967).

* denotes subjective side-effects.

With such techniques at hand it also becomes possible to carry out biologically-oriented experiments within the framework of a clinical trial. This has been done by Elkes who has tested the hypothesis that depressive patients who respond to desmethylimipramine metabolise the drug more slowly than those who do not, thereby giving the drug more time to exert its pharmaco-dynamic action (Elkes, 1968). It would follow from this hypothesis that unresponsive patients should excrete larger amounts of unchanged drug, there being more of it to excrete, than patients who are responsive to desmethylimipramine. On this assumption Elkes proceeded to employ the general structure and criteria of the M.R.C. trial of the treatment of depressive illness in order, first, to eliminate placebo-responders and then to make comparative biochemical observations on those patients who did and did not respond to medication. The rate of metabolism of desmethylimipramine was studied by fluorimetric measurement of the percentage of the daily dose excreted in a 24-hour specimen of urine; in addition, thin-layer chromatography made it possible to display the metabolites of desmethylimipramine and estimate their relative quantities in urine. In the event Elkes' results appear to be negative, in that no clear-cut difference emerged between responders but experiments of this type may confidently be expected to extend the scope of clinical trials of anti-depressants as biological methods become more refined.

3. In addition to clinical and biological variables, however, account must also be taken of the influence of social factors on the apparent response to pharmacotherapy. Such factors have been shown to bear on discharge from hospital, which is often taken as an index of amelioration (Watt and Buglass, 1966). Among such factors marital status is of indisputable importance. Patients with depression are known to enter hospital earlier and stay longer if they are single than if they are married. Further, Angst has claimed that this relationship remains demonstrable after treatment with anti-depressants (Angst, 1965). We may hope to see this dimension further explored in the evaluation of these drugs in future.

The prophylaxis of depression

The notion of prevention has recently become prominent in the literature on anti-depressant medication and is likely to grow in volume. It is implicit in the rationale of 'maintenance' therapy, which is the subject of a current M.R.C. investigation, but much of the discussion so far has been focussed on lithium carbonate following the claim that it is 'the first drug for which a clear-cut prophylactic action against one of the major psychoses has been demonstrated' (Baastrup and Schou, 1967). The fallacies in the logic of this claim have been pointed out elsewhere (Blackwell and Shepherd, 1968) but the prospect of preventing depression by chemical means has already proved irresistible in some centres and, in the process, has even resulted in a challenge to the proper use of clinical trials. Thus, in Sweden a double-blind study has been terminated for 'ethical' reasons on the following grounds:

'From the start we decided not to include patients with severe affective psychoses—i.e. with very frequent relapses, serious suicidal attempts, and/or long social disablement. These patients were instead assigned to an " open " lithium group, on the grounds that, although Dr. Baastrup and Dr. Schou may not have afforded proof of the prophylactic action of lithium, they have nevertheless provided so much evidence that we felt it unethical to deprive severely ill patients of this chance. Since we formed the impression that patients in this open lithium group reacted favourably, and since colleagues from other hospitals reported similar consistent impressions, our unwillingness to deprive patients of lithium increased. From at first excluding only the graver cases, we gradually allowed even milder cases to join the open lithium group, which meant that fewer cases became available for the double-blind study.

'Another cause of the failure of the experiment was the publicity that lithium has been given in Sweden, where most psychiatrists believe that its value far outweighs its risks in severe recurrent affective psychoses. Our patients got to know that lithium was considered to have a prophylactic effect, and several of them specifically asked for it. We have known most of our patients for several years; they apply to the clinic when they have a relapse, and thus it was not easy to include them in a double-blind study. In our opinion, it is now too late to make a study in Sweden in which a simultaneous control group is not given lithium. The problem might be less in countries where knowledge of lithium is more limited or the psychological conditions different' (Laurell and Ottosson, 1968).

Such a viewpoint backed up by the asseveration that ' observer bias and psychological factors are probably not major sources of error ', would seem to bring us back to our point of departure, namely the importance of attitudes adopted to clinical trials. Perhaps I may be permitted to conclude by not only deprecating the attitude exemplified by the foregoing quotation but by reaffirming what I wrote 10 years ago: ' It now seems probable that we are soon to be presented with so many new anti-depressive compounds that the familiar clinical attitude of laissez-faire empiricism will be increasingly difficult to sustain. The clinician is compelled to hold the balance between the scales of laboratory data on the one hand and stochastic theory on the other. Though his experience and judgement are essential it will be necessary for him to adopt a more experimental role in the future if he is to co-operate fully with the pharmacologist and the statistician, whose techniques he should understand if full weight is to be given to observations made in the clinical setting. More clinical research is indispensable to progress in the evaluation of drugs for the treatment of depression '.

I would predict that these comments are likely to be still more applicable to the seventies than they have been to the sixties.

REFERENCES

ANGST, J. (1965). Erfolg und Misserfolg der psychopharmakologischen Therapie am Beispiel der Depression. *Hippokrates,* **36,** 946.

BAASTRUP, P. C. & SCHOU, M. (1967). Lithium as a prophylactic agent. *Archs Gen. Psychiat.* **16,** 162.

BLACKWELL, B. & SHEPHERD, M. (1967). Early evaluation of psychotropic drugs in man. *Lancet,* **2,** 819.

BLACKWELL, B. & SHEPHERD, M. (1968). Prophylactic lithium: another therapeutic myth? *Lancet,* **1,** 968.

BRODIE, B. B. (1965). Some ideas on the mode of action of imipramine-type antidepressants. In *The Scientific Basis of Drug Therapy in Psychiatry,* ed. Marks, J. & Pare, C. M. B., p. 127. Oxford: Pergamon Press.

ELKES, A. (1968). Mode of action of imipramine. *M.D. Thesis,* University of London.

HAMMER, W. & SJÖQVIST, F. (1967). Plasma levels of monomethylated tricyclic antidepressants during treatment with imipramine-like compounds. *Life Sci.* **6,** 1895.

KENDELL, R. E. (1968). The problem of classification. In *Recent Developments in Affective Disorders,* ed. Coppen, A. & Walk, A. *Br. J. Psychiat.* Special Publiction No. 2. p. 15. Headley Bros. Ltd.

KIMBELL, I., OVERALL, J. E. & HOLLISTER, J. E. (1965). Antidepressant drugs: myth or reality? *J. New Drugs,* **5,** 9.

LAURELL, B. & OTTOSSON, J. O. (1968). Prophylactic lithium? *Lancet,* **2,** 1245.

LEYBURN, P. (1967). A critical look at antidepressant drug trials. *Lancet,* **2,** 1135.

MEDICAL RESEARCH COUNCIL (1965). (Report by its Clinical Committee.) Clinical trial of the treatment of depressive illness. *Br. med. J.* **1,** 881.

SHEPHERD, M. (1959). Evaluation of drugs in the treatment of depression. *Can. psychiat. Ass. J.* Special Suppl. **4,** S120.

SHEPHERD, M. (1967a). Implications of a multi-centred clinical trial of treatments of depressive illness. In *Anti-depressant Drugs,* ed. Garattini, S. & Dukes, M. N. G. p. 332. Amsterdam: Excerpta Medica.

SHEPHERD, M. (1967b). The method of the multi-centred clinical trial. In *Neuropsychopharmacology,* ed. Brill, H., Cole, J. O., Deniker, P., Hippius, H. & Bradley, P. B. p. 51. Amsterdam: Excerpta Medica.

SJÖQVIST, F., HAMMER, W., IDESTROM, C-M., LIND, M., TUCK, D. & ÅSBERG, M. (1968). Plasma level of monomethylated tricyclic antidepressants and side-effects in man. In *Proceedings of the European Society for the Study of Drug Toxicity.* Vol. IX, Toxicity and Side-effects of Psychotropic Drugs. p. 246. Amsterdam: Excerpta Medica.

SLOANE, R. B. (1959). Discussion (of paper by Shepherd, M.). *Can. psychiat. Ass. J.* Special Suppl. **4,** S.126.

WATT, D. C. & BUGLASS, D. (1966). The effect of clinical and social factors on the discharge of chronic psychiatric patients. *Soc. Psychiat.* **1,** 57.

WECHSLER, H., GROSSER, G. H. & GREENSBLATT, M. (1965). Research evaluating antidepressant medications on hospitalised mental patients. *J. nerv. ment. Dis.* **141,** 231.

WORLD HEALTH ORGANIZATION (1967). Research in psychopharmacology. *Tech. Rep. Ser. Wld Hlth Org.* No. 371.

EVALUATION OF PSYCHOTROPIC DRUGS

(3) SEDATIVES

M. HAMILTON

Introduction

Other papers in this symposium have dealt with various problems of drug trials in a general way. They are: definition of clinical condition, clarification of questions to be answered, certain practical difficulties and the methods of coping with them and, finally, the measurement of the criterion. This one will deal with these problems in terms of the use of sedatives for the treatment of anxiety. The aim of treatment, and therefore of a clinical trial, is the amelioration of a pathological or abnormal state, which is defined in terms either of target symptoms, a pattern or group of symptoms, or of a syndrome or disorder. Examples of target symptoms are tension, palpitations, headache or insomnia. They occur very commonly in groups, e.g. indigestion, frequency of micturition, palpitations, sweating and headaches are typical of the somatic symptoms of anxiety. Symptoms such as tension, insomnia, continuous apprehension, forgetfulness and irritability are examples of associated symptoms at the level of behaviour (psychological level).

Finally, as a syndrome or disorder we talk of a condition known as ' anxiety state ' or ' anxiety neurosis '.

Target symptoms are easy to define but they do not exist in isolation; they normally manifest themselves as part of a pattern of biological activity at the physiological and behavioural level. To confine a trial to a consideration of just one is therefore too narrow an aim. In any case the assessment of one symptom is too unreliable for most purposes. A much better approach is to consider groups of symptoms. Empirically, it is known from their intercorrelations that they do in fact occur in groups. Furthermore, sufficient is known about the mechanisms underlying them to indicate a functional unity for certain groups (not necessarily the same as the groups found by methods of correlation). Finally, the alteration of functions due to the effect of drugs is sometimes related to these particular mechanisms. It is of interest that drug trials in the U.S.A. tend to concentrate on target symptoms or groups of symptoms, whereas in the United Kingdom, they concentrate more on the amelioration of ' anxiety state '.

Anxiety states and their diagnosis

The term ' anxiety state ' or ' anxiety neurosis ' is intended to delineate a disorder, but the outlines of this are not at all clear.

Different schools of psychiatry use the term differently and subdivide the general term differently. For example, in Europe it is common to refer to ' vegetative dystonia ' which is a sub-division of the affective disorders similar to but not entirely the same as anxiety state. A good paper should define the condition clearly and indicate which sort of patients are excluded and included in the trial. This is not often done. There are two reasons for this; the first is that writers in technical journals are reluctant to define elementary notions which they believe are known to all readers and the second is that for reasons of economy of space, editors are apt to frown severely upon those who waste it on ' unnecessary ' detail.

The difficulties in defining anxiety states are found on two aspects. In the first, there is the difficulty of distinguishing between a patient with an anxious disposition who has a high reactivity (or low thresh-hold) to stress, from one who is suffering from a pathological state. Such persons constantly experience circumstances which increase their anxiety, sometimes to a level at which they feel the need for treatment. Since such exacerbations are usually of a temporary nature, and in any case fluctuate continually, it is not easy to define what is meant by ' treatment ' in the usual sense. Clinical trials usually exclude such individuals and concern themselves with patients who are suffering from an actual pathological condition. This begs the question as to whether there is in fact a real difference between the pathological state and the exaggerated form of the anxious personality. Some schools of psychiatry believe that there is no difference and all distinctions are quite arbitrary.

The other aspect is concerned with the problem of distinguishing between those patients who are suffering from an anxiety state and who complain also of depressed mood, and those who are suffering from a depressive illness which is accompanied by anxiety. This is the condition sometimes referred to as ' reactive ' or ' neurotic ' depression. Recent work has shown that this particular problem is more complicated than had previously been thought. Black (1966) in a study of the placebo response suggested that his findings indicated that ' anxiety states ' were not a homogeneous group. Hays (1964) showed that a typical depressive illness could be preceded sometimes by a prodromal period, lasting up to several years, of mild symptoms of chronic anxiety. Snaith (1968) pointed out that patients suffering from anxiety states may have recurrent clear-cut episodes with intervening periods free from symptoms; this is the characteristic feature of the manic-depressive disorders. Walker (1959) described a group of patients, diagnosed as suffering from anxiety states which were characterised by a sudden onset of symptoms and episodes of tension without precipitant factors. These patients all had a uniformly good prognosis and he suggested that they were ' really ' depressive states. Thus, many patients suffering from ' anxiety states ' show features which clearly resemble those of the affective disorders, even of the manic-depressive type. From the other direction, Carney *et al.* (1965) in their studies on the depressions, in relation to classification and response to ECT, described ' neurotic depressions' in such a way that they are very difficult to distinguish from anxiety states.

All this work is still very recent and has not yet been assimilated into the general body of accepted psychiatric knowledge. Hence it is ignored in current drug trials. There can be no doubt that if these studies are confirmed there will have to be a re-evaluation of all previous work in this field, even for drug trials confined to symptomatic improvement of target or grouped symptoms. This must be so because it cannot be assumed that the same symptom, occurring in different settings, will respond always in the same manner to a given treatment.

Clarification of questions in a trial

Many of the problems which cause difficulty in drug trials in other mental disorders are of little importance when we are dealing with the use of sedatives for the treatment of anxiety. One of the more important ones is the differentiation between short- and long-term effects of treatment. Very little work has been done on the long-term effects of continuous medication and most trials confine themselves to the effect of treatment for a period of two to three months at most. The rate of improvement is of little importance in this field, since most drugs are quite quick-acting, though other difficulties can arise here. If the criterion of improvement consists of the patient's subjective impression of amelioration of his symptoms, there will always be a bias in favour of quick-acting drugs as against slow-acting ones. There are some drug trials, often quoted in the literature, which suffer from this defect and have not taken it into account. The safety of drugs is an important consideration in modern drug trials and as a result, present-day sedatives are very much safer than older ones. On the other hand, side-effects are a problem which have not yet been solved. It can be said still that, by and large, efficacy and side-effects are closely linked.

Criterion of improvement

The criterion of improvement can be conveniently subdivided into four categories: subjective and objective changes, personal relations and working capacity. Subjective improvement is concerned with a patient's own feelings, whereas objective improvement is concerned with his behaviour. For example, tension and inability to relax can be regarded as the subjective aspect of the objective behaviour found in outbursts of temper. The relation between these two aspects is close but not so close that there is no point in differentiating between them; in any case, the methods of assessment do differ. Furthermore, the difference between subjective and objective assessment may show itself quite radically because of problems of threshold. Thus, a patient suffering from anxiety state who has difficulty in going out of doors because of the increasing anxiety that this produces (agoraphobia) may show a subjective diminution of anxiety and yet still not be able to go out of doors. On the other hand his improvement may show itself as an ability to go out of doors, and yet he himself may complain that his anxiety is not much diminished. All four types of criterion are positively correlated, but it is worth considering them separately. Most drug trials concentrate on subjective and objective improvement, probably because it is easy to measure by present techniques, but there is no doubt that the criteria of improvement in personal relations and improvement in working capacity are very important and it would be highly desirable to place greater emphasis on these in the future.

Practical problems

'*Suggestibility.*' The most difficult of the practical problems is ' suggestibility ' or ' placebo response ', the rapid improvement that occurs in anxious patients under any therapeutic regime. This may arise from the feelings of security and comfort produced merely by being seen by a physician who understands the patient's symptoms; but the therapist may do more, from reassurance and explanation up to some form of simple psychotherapy. The improvement due to suggestibility will obviously tend to hide the effects of additional treatment, i.e. drugs. Most trials depend upon the fact that non-specific improvement takes place rapidly and soon tails off. Hence, a trial which lasts longer than three weeks will tend to minimise the relative effect of suggestion, but, of course, it cannot eliminate it, for it will still make a major contribution to the improvement in both treated and controlled groups. Some drug trials have attempted to cope with this problem, e.g. Kellner *et al.* (1968) allowed a ' practice ' week and then made the first assessment of the patient. Hargreaves *et al.* (1958) allowed a period of two weeks before making a first assessment for the trial. Roberts and Hamilton (1958) examined the improvement in detail and found that anxious mood, insomnia and tension improved significantly in these two weeks. Subsequently it was found, by examining the changes in the group of patients receiving placebo during the course of the trial, that there was an improvement in autonomic and general somatic symptoms. To cope with this non-specific improvement, it would be advisable to make baseline assessments for the initial period of the trial at about two weeks and four weeks and to look for drug-effects after this.

'*Habituation.*' Habituation to drugs varies considerably, but there is no doubt about its existence in sedatives. It is fairly rapid in onset as recent researches have shown, and can be valuable. For example, patients may complain of being sleepy when they are first given a sedative, or an anti-depressive, but this diminishes within a week or two. Unfortunately, such side symptoms may lead to patients abandoning their treatment or decreasing the dose they take. One way of dealing with this is to start with a very small dose and work up to an adequate dose slowly, but this, of course, leads to a lengthening of the trial. In general, habituation gives rise to difficulties in the reverse direction in that it tends to diminish the effect of a sedative. The real difficulty here arises from the possibility of transfer effects: patients have already been on other sedatives and have become habituated to them and this tends to diminish their responsiveness to the new drug under trial. Such transfer effects have been little studied and this is to be regretted because it is rare for patients not to have received sedative drugs before they come on to a trial. The problem of a transfer-effect arising from the consumption of alcohol also needs to be considered. The phenomenon of habituation is of fundamental importance in relation to cross-over trials and this is one of the reasons why they should be regarded with some suspicion.

'*Variables affecting response.*' On the whole, insufficient attention has been paid to extraneous factors which affect the response to drugs or the conduct of a trial. For example, Black (1966) found that there was a greater placebo response in patients with a history of illness of less than one year. The interaction between sedatives and psychotherapy has also been insufficiently investigated, though at least one paper is worth studying in this connection—Lorr *et al.* (1963). One paper which considered the effect of extraneous factors on drug action is that by Ward and Parsonage (1961). This was an elegant little trial on the effects of Methylpentynol for reducing anxiety during the taking of EEGs. The trial was designed as a factorial experiment:

drugs X sex X technician

The active drug was compared with a placebo, the data for men and women were kept distinct and the experiment was conducted under two conditions, i.e. two EEG technicians were compared, since they were very different personalities and coped with the patients in very different ways. Assessment was by means of self-rating, clinical rating and EEG changes. It was found that with the last there was a clear significant interaction between the drugs and sex, which means that the effect of the drugs was different in the two sexes. An important paper which illustrates these problems is that by Reynolds *et al.* (1965). In very many ways, this paper is a text-book example on how to conduct drug trials. For example, an important pre-treatment check was carried out; after randomisation, the groups of patients were tested to see whether they were comparable. Furthermore, the results obtained by the two physicians who did the clinical work were compared. In both cases significant differences were found and were considered in relation to the results of the trial. It is impossible to over-emphasise the importance of such examination of the data. Although, strictly speaking, it is illegitimate to do so *post hoc,* such differences can sometimes be eliminated by co-variance, or by stratification or both. It is true that this makes the statistical analysis difficult but then that is what computers are for.

Measurement of criterion

Self rating scales. Self rating scales offer a great convenience in that they save the time of the physician in making assessments and they can be repeated frequently. They are particularly useful in evaluating drugs for the treatment of anxiety, because the usual contraindications are more or less irrelevant; for example, the patients are too ill to fill them in, the patients cannot understand them or the scale includes states that cannot be perceived by the patient, such as retardation or hypochondriasis. Nevertheless, they are still liable to bias and this should be taken into account before deciding to use them. The number of such scales is slowly increasing and it is to be hoped that the following brief review will help in making a choice.

The Maudsley Personality Inventory (1959) and its more recent version, the Eysenck Personality Inventory (1964) are easy to administer, have been extensively used and have norms for the general population. It differentiates well between neurotics and normals but is not sensitive to drug effects, e.g. Robinson *et al.* (1965). This may be related to the fact that it is supposed to measure ' neuroticism ' rather than anxiety as such, i.e. to measure characteristics of personality rather than a temporary fluctuating state. Taylor's Manifest Anxiety Scale (1953) is derived from the M.M.P.I. and consists of a number of items printed on cards which have to be classified by the patient as true, false or query. It has been very much used in drug trials, though there has been some criticism of its value. Kellner *et al.* (1968) found it insensitive to the differences between an active drug and placebo. The active drug had been found to show significant differences by other methods of assessment. However, when these authors scored the M.A.S. as a check list (counting the positive items) they found that it did show some significant difference between drug and placebo, but it was the least useful of all the methods of assessment used in their enquiry. The Heineman Anxiety Scale (1953) is essentially a form of the Taylor M.A.S. given by the method of ' forced choice '. I have not been able to find whether it has been used in drug trials, but it ought to be considered from the point of view of helping to diminish problems of bias. The Costello and Comrey Scale for Anxiety (1967) is a self-rating scale which has been recently developed and thoroughly tested. It clearly differentiates between neurotics and normals and has been very carefully designed to eliminate bias in answering questions due to the social desirability or undesirability of items. For example, subjects and patients are reluctant to answer affirmatively to such statements as ' I am awkward with members of the opposite sex ', and ' I am bad tempered '. The elimination of such bias signifies that this scale is likely to be a great improvement on the M.A.S. but it has not been used in drug trials so far as I know.

Cattell's I.P.A.T. Anxiety Scale (Cattell and Scheier, 1957) is a well-known scale but was developed, as most of Cattell's scales, chiefly for use with normal subjects; I have found only one trial which used this scale (Robinson *et al.*, 1965) and those investigators came to the conclusion that the I.P.A.T. Scale was unsatisfactory but it must be admitted that it was not given a fair test. It was used in a trial comparing oxypertine versus placebo and was unable to distinguish between the two. On the other hand, no differences between the two treatments were found with either of the other two scales used, both of which have been regarded as satisfactory in the sense of being capable of demonstrating drug effects.

The Anxiety Scale published by Gleser *et al.* (1961) is ingenious and very different from others. The patient is asked to talk about his life or important events in his life for a period of five minutes. This is tape-recorded and typed out and the speech is analysed by a special method described by the authors. It is laborious to score but it has obvious advantages in that it does not ask for deliberate judgements to be made by the patient. It might be of use in drug trials under some circumstances.

Rating scales by observers. One of the most well-known of rating scales is the Brief Psychiatric Rating Scale (B.P.R.S.) of Overall and Gorham (1962). It is a general all-purpose scale for all psychiatric symptoms. It has been extensively used and well validated and, above all, has been shown to be sensitive to drug response. From the present point of view it is probably not very satisfactory as only 3 out of the 16 items are directly related to anxiety. A new form has been developed, the Factor Construct Rating Scale (F.C.R.S.). This is an improvement on the other from the present point of view, in that although it contains only three out of 17 items directly related to anxiety, another 4 are indirectly related. The Symptom Rating Test (S.R.T.) of Kellner and Sheffield (1968) consists of a semi-structured interview, based on a check list of neurotic symptoms, which is then followed by the self rating of each symptom on three scales: intensity, frequency and duration. It differentiates well between neurotics and normals and is sensitive to changes during treatment. Kellner *et al.* (1968) found it very sensitive to drug effects. Another form consists of a self-rating scale of 40 items, each rated on a four-point scale.

The rating scale of Buss *et al.* (1955) is a well-designed scale for covering observed behaviour and subjective symptoms. It has a high correlation with the Taylor M.A.S. It is intended to be used for rating a patient's condition at the time of interview and is not suitable for a ' present state ' covering, for example, a week because of the items dealing with ' observed behaviour '. I have not been able to discover any drug trials which have used this and I suspect it has been unjustly neglected. It bears some resemblance to the rating scale for anxiety states of Hamilton (1959). This is a rating scale for assessment of symptoms of the patient in general, i.e. covering a recent period of time, despite one item ' Behaviour at interview '. It is intended for use by psychiatrists and other skilled observers. Compared with the scale of Buss *et al.* it gives a greater weight to somatic symptoms; of the 13 items, 6 are devoted to the physical symptoms of anxiety. Robinson *et al.* (1965) used 11 items in a drug trial and found it very satisfactory. They found that two observers had a disagreement of only plus or minus one point for between 66 and 93 per cent patients ($N=29$). In the paper by Kellner *et al.* (1968) mentioned above, it was found to be the most sensitive of the various scales used in this trial, showing the maximum difference between active and inactive drugs.

These last two papers are extremely valuable because the investigators used more than one scale for examining the effects of drugs in a trial. Only in this way can the value of scales be determined. It would be highly desirable if other investigators would follow their example.

Physiological measures

The last few years have seen the appearance of physiological measures for measuring anxiety and this is a development which is highly to be desired. What hampers their spread at the moment is the lack of equipment and, above all, skilled users. In this connection the monograph of Lader and Wing (1966) deserves careful study. A new method, forearm plethysmography, has been developed by Kelly (1967). Compared with other methods it is a fairly simple one. The first attempts to validate it could be improved upon. Kelly and Walter (1968) found that basal forearm blood flow was higher in 41 patients suffering from chronic anxiety states than in 60 normal controls and this difference was highly significant statistically. The correlation with Taylor's M.A.S. was ·21, but this is of no interest in the present context, as the M.A.S. is not sensitive to changes in anxiety. Further work will have to be done on this psycho-physiological technique; its future looks very promising.

Summary

A review of the literature shows that in recent years standards of clinical trials of sedatives have improved considerably. Closer attention has been paid to factors relating to the effects of treatment. Unfortunately, not enough have used variable dosage of drugs and too many still use the method of cross-over trials. New work on the nature of anxiety states will lead to finer sub-division of this group. The improvement in defining the types of patients involved in trials will therefore make clearer the indications for different treatments.

Improvements in measuring the criteria may be expected, in the development of new rating scales and new self-assessment questionnaires. Finally, the development of physiological methods will undoubtedly improve the measurement of the criteria in this field; but it must not be forgotten that physiological methods will always need to be validated against clinical assessment, at least in the first instance, and also under specific conditons for particular drugs.

REFERENCES

BLACK, A. A. (1966). Factors predisposing to a placebo response in new out-patients with anxiety states. *Br. J. Psychiat.* **112,** 557.

BUSS, A. H., WIENER, M., DURKEE, A. & BAER, M. (1955). The measurement of anxiety in clinical situations. *J. consult. Psychol.* **19,** 125.

CARNEY, M. W. P., ROTH, M. & GARSIDE, R. F. (1965). The diagnosis of depressive syndromes and the prediction of E.C.T. response. *Br. J. Psychiat.* **111,** 659.

CATTELL, R. B. & SCHEIER, I. H. (1957). *IPAT Anxiety Scale.* Illinois: Champagne.

COSTELLO, C. G. & COMREY, A. L. ((1967). Scales for measuring depression and anxiety. *J. Psychol.* **66,** 303.

EYSENCK, H. J. (1959). *Manual of the Maudsley Personality Inventory.* London: University of London Press.

EYSENCK, H. J. & EYSENCK, S. B. G. (1964). *Manual of the Eysenck Personality Inventory.* London: University of London Press.

GLESER, C. G., GOTTSCHALK, L. A. & SPRINGER, K. J. (1961). An anxiety scale applicable to verbal samples. *Arch. gen. Psychiat.* **5,** 593.

HAMILTON, M. (1959). The assessment of anxiety states by rating. *Br. J. med. Psychol.* **32,** 50.

HARGREAVES, G. R., HAMILTON, M. & ROBERTS, J. M. (1958). Clinical trial of benactyzine in anxiety states. *J. ment. Sci.* **104,** 1056.

HAYS, P. (1964). Modes of onset of psychotic depression. *Br. med. J.* **2,** 779.

HEINEMAN, C. E. (1953). A forced-choice form of the Taylor Anxiety Scale. *J. consult. Psychol.* **17,** 447.

KELLNER, R., KELLY, A. V. & SHEFFIELD, B. F. (1968). The assessment of changes in anxiety in a drug trial: a comparison of methods. *Br. J. Psychiat.* **114,** 863.

KELLNER, R. & SHEFFIELD, B. F. (1968). The use of self-rating scales in a single patient multiple cross-over trial. *Br. J. Psychiat.* **114,** 193.

KELLY, D. H. W. (1967). The technique of forearm plethysmography for assessing anxiety. *J. psychosom. Res.* **10,** 373.

KELLY, D. H. W. & WALTER, C. J. S. (1968). The relationship between clinical diagnosis and anxiety, assessed by forearm blood flow and other measurements. *Br. J. Psychiat.* **114,** 611.

LADER, M. H. & WING, L. (1966). Physiological measures, sedative drugs and morbid anxiety. *Maudsley Monograph No. 14.* London: Chapman and Hall.

LORR, M., MCNAIR, D. M. & WEINSTEIN, G. L. (1963). Early effects of chlordiazepoxide (Librium) used with psychotherapy. *J. psychiat. Res.* **1,** 257.

OVERALL, J. E. & GORHAM, G. R. (1962). The Brief Psychiatric Rating Scale. *Psychol. Rep.* **10,** 799.

ROBERTS, J. M. & HAMILTON, M. (1958). The effects of suggestion on the symptoms of anxiety states. *J. ment. Sci.* **104,** 1052.

REYNOLDS, E., JOYCE, C. R. B., SWIFT, J. L., TOOLEY, P. H. & WETHERALL, M. (1965). Psychological and clinical investigation of the treatment of anxiety out-patients with three barbiturates and placebo. *Br. J. Psychiat.* **111,** 84.

ROBINSON, J. T., DAVIES, L. S., KREITMAN, N. & KNOWLES, J. B. (1965). A double-blind trial of oxypertine for anxiety neurosis. *Br. J. Psychiat.* **111**, 527.

SNAITH, R. P. (1968). A clinical investigation of phobias. *Br. J. Psychiat.* **114**, 673.

TAYLOR, J. A. (1953). A personality scale of manifest anxiety. *J. abnorm. soc. Psychol.* **48**, 285.

WALKER, L. (1959). The prognosis for affective illness with overt anxiety. *J. Neurol. Neurosurg. Psychiat.* **22**, 338.

WARD, B. & PARSONAGE, M. J. (1961). A controlled factorial trial of the use of methylpentynol in the short term reduction of anxiety during EEG examination. *Acta psychiat. scand.* **37**, 331.

HOW TO IMPROVE AT CLINICAL TRIALS

C. R. B. JOYCE

How many clinical trials do we need to test the efficacy of new drugs? And how many trialists? If there is only one indication for the use of each new drug (a conservative assumption), we shall surely ask for a minimum of three trials per drug (results must be reproducible, and the number must be odd, on the committee principle, in case of dissension). If about 50 new drugs come on the market each year and if each of these is the survivor of 20 that the Medical Advisers have put out to trial, there will have to be 3,000 trials per year. Since, in our own experience as well as others', each trial runs for an average of about two years at least, 6,000 trials will be going on at any one time. Mainland suggests (1960) that it is a full-time job for a controller to run three trials at once. (Our own small-scale experience confirms this: in 10 years we have undertaken 24 trials—of which, incidentally, we initiated four, drug companies eight, and our colleagues the remainder: four were not proceeded with after preliminary discussion, three terminated early, 12 have been completed and are the subject of 15 papers. On average, two members of the department spent rather less than half their total research time on the organisation of clinical trials.)

Consequently, it seems as if we need *at least* 2,000 people who are skilful enough to control (i.e., design, run and analyse) trials; and that, since 10 years' hard labour of this kind is an adequate preparation for early retirement to an insane asylum, we need to be training at least 200 replacements a year. Who should they be? How should they be trained?

This paper briefly describes one answer to the second question. The answer to the first is even briefer. It is: 'Anyone—provided that he doesn't come into direct contact with the patients.' A trial controller need not be medically qualified; he need not in fact be a statistician, since the planning of a trial must be a corporate affair, the design of which can be worked out by a consultant surgeon, a psychiatrist or a ward orderly, if they have the necessary skills (the latter quite often have, especially during summer vacations). The controller's main tasks have been described elsewhere (Joyce, 1968): for the present purpose, the emphasis is on the necessity for him to convert the design, if it is not his own, to a ' blind ' form.

If one were being unduly cynical, one would say that the only thing ever learnt from a clinical trial is not how to improve at the next trial design but how one might have done the last one better. Each poses its own problems; no two are ever the same; even a hack replication never is—there are inevitable staff changes and in a replication the problem of morale becomes even more important, if possible, than usual. However, there is some transfer of training and some generalisation is possible. But to an extent that surprises those who suppose that clinical trials are the nearest thing in clinical medicine to the exercise of hard scientific method, what has to be learnt has a good deal of art in it and can therefore be learnt only in the execution.

Or in the simulation of an execution: and for those who are lazy, hard up for hardware, or both, simulation does not necessarily involve the use of a computer. It is true that a computer trial simulation, though it will involve, even for a small trial, an enormous amount of data generation and contingency programming, will allow the individual student to make his own mistakes and to ask his own questions. But our cheap and lazy method has the advantage that it uses group discussion as the basic unit of training, and so gives increased opportunities for everyone, especially the group leaders, to learn from each other.

The method is very simple. It only requires the running protocols kept from the inception to completion of one clinical trial, though in more detail than is usually the case, but not in more detail than should be the case, together with the clinical observations arising in the course of it.

CLINICAL TRIAL SIMULATION DOCUMENTS

No.	Document	Issued
1	The problem	Pre-course
2	Primary objectives	First session
3	Criteria for admission Criteria for exclusion	First session
4	Detailed procedure	Second session
5	Clinical proforma	Second session
6	Logistics	Second session
7	Design	Second session
8	Intended analyses	Second session
9	Clinical observations	Third session
10	Patients' and doctors' preferences	Third session
11	Analyses—non-parametric	Final session
12	Analyses—parametric	Final session
13	What else went wrong?	
	1. that we discovered	Final session
	2. that we were told	Final session
14	Chronology	Final session
15	Evaluation	Post-course
16	Bibliography	Post-course

Fig. 1

The categories of information from the successive stages in one such trial are shown in Figure 1. We used this method with some 50 participants in a two-day training workshop in association with the Trust for Education and Research in Therapeutics. The students were told the general object of the trial at the time of their enrolment, namely ' To compare reserpine and guanethidine in symptomless previously untreated hypertension '. I do not intend to explain here why we thought it necessary, starting in August 1965, to carry out such a trial; Dr Dunne (this volume, page 235) deals to some extent with such metaphysical questions. The participants were also asked to consider, before the course began, how they would frame the ' primary objectives ' of such a trial.

The course members were allocated to one of four groups, each of which was jointly led by two experienced trialists, one from the Department of Pharmacology and Therapeutics, London Hospital Medical College, and one medical adviser to the pharmaceutical industry. The composition of each group was balanced as far as possible in terms of the provenance of its members but ' streamed ' for previous experience of trials in the light of answers—which were certainly far too modest—to a pre-course questionnaire. There were four small group discussions, each lasting between 60 and 90 minutes, separated by more formal contributions from some of the leaders on such technical aspects as programming, the use of lector forms, nonparametric tests, etc. Most course members would have liked more of these; there was complete agreement that there should have been more discussion periods.

Each discussion was introduced by the leader putting the problem to be discussed to the participants, who then worked out their own solution to it before the leader revealed the ' solution ' (frequently less satisfactory) adopted in the actual trial, in the form of a printed hand-out. As can be seen from Figure 1, there was frequently more than one discussion in each discussion period: for example, the primary objectives (Fig. 2) and criteria for admission to and exclusion from the trial (Fig. 3) were both discussed in the first session.

PRIMARY OBJECTIVES

1. Comparison of low doses of guanethidine and reserpine on moderately elevated blood pressure
2. Incidence of unwanted actions
3. Patient and doctor preferences for each drug
4. Relation of treatment outcome to social and psychological factors in individual patients
5. Assessment of patient coop eration by pill returns and (possibly) urine tests

FIG. 2

The discussions, in fact, followed in the compressed time of a few hours the three years or so (Fig. 4) that the real trial had taken. At any time the academic leaders, three of whom had been involved in some capacity in the trial, could be asked for information not on the hand-outs and could usually provide it from their own knowledge. The only constraint, and an admittedly serious one from the educational point of view, was that the decisions of the group or the opinions of an individual member could in no way modify the progress of the trial. Some compensation for this lack of servo-control was obtained from a final hand-out detailing 'What else went wrong?' (Fig. 5). This covered aspects that we know about; Dr Dunne also deals with some errors that we only suspected.

CRITERIA FOR SELECTION

1. Either sex
2. Under 45 years of age
3. Diastolic > 90 mm on first attendance
4. No previous treatment for hypertension

EXCLUSIONS

1. Malignant hypertension
2. Diabetes mellitus
3. Evidence of cardiac, cerebral or renal damage from hypertension or atheroma

FIG. 3

CHRONOLOGY

Stage	Date	Time elapsed (months)
Conception	17. 8.1965	0
First meeting	7.11.1965	2.5
First schedule prepared	17.11.1965	3.0
Dummy run	1.12.1965	3.5
Revised schedule prepared	23. 2.1966	6.0
Forms prepared	22. 6.1966	10.0
Drugs received	23. 6.1966	10.0
First patient admitted	24. 8.1966	12.0
Last (35th) patient admitted	21. 9.1967	25.0
Last (32nd) patient made choice	2. 5.1968	31.5
Code broken and analysis started	2. 5.1968	31.5
Report finished	31.12.1968	39.5
Report accepted	14. 2.1969	41.0
Report published		

FIG. 4

WHAT ELSE WENT WRONG?

1. 90 G.Ps. circulated; only 9 referred patients
2. About half the patients referred did not conform to criteria
3. Admission criteria too restrictive; age limit (45) relaxed
4. Required frequency of visits a strain on working, symptomless patients
5. Lector forms often not completed in clinic
6. Objectives of social survey not specific enough
7. Period of placebo treatment useful
8. Several patients gave misleading pill returns. Satisfactory chemical tests for blood and urine concentrations required
9. Leakage of information on treatments to physicians from Pharmacy?
10. Etc.

FIG. 5

FORM NO.	PAGE NUMBER	(iii)...(ii)...(i)...	10	6	3 2	1
NO. OF PATIENT IN TRIAL	BRANCH NUMBER	60 30 20 10		6	3 2	1
DAY	WEEK NUMBER	30 20 10		6	3 2	1
MONTH	600 300 200 100 JAN...FEB...MAR...APR	60 30 20 10 MAY...JUN...JUL...AUG		6 3 2 1 SEP...OCT...NOV...DEC		
YEAR						
HOSPITAL NO. xxx.. ..						
xx ..						
.. xx						
TRIAL PHASE (PREVIOUS PERIOD)		SPARE		1A...1B...2...3		
DURATION OF PHASE (WEEKS)	600 300 200 100	60 30 20 10		6 3 2 1		
INTERVAL SINCE LAST SEEN (WEEKS)	DEFAULT	REFER				
MEDICATION TAKEN SINCE LAST VISIT	CODE NO A... B...	DAILY DOSE TABLETS		NO. DOSES/DAY		
NO. OF TABLETS TAKEN	FEW ... MOST	ALL				
OTHER MEDICATIONS TAKEN	YES ... NO	REFER				

SYMPTOMS SINCE LAST VISIT

	HEADACHE	EPISTAXIS	OTHR REFER NONE
PERSISTENT H.T.	+ ++	+ ++	
CARDIOVASCULAR COMPLICATIONS	ORTHOPNOEA + ++ CHEST PAIN (EXERCISE) + ++	ANKLE SWELLING + ++ CHEST PAIN AT REST + ++	OTHR REFER NONE
NEUROLOGICAL COMPLICATIONS	SPEECH + ++ VISUAL + ++	WEAKNESS + ++ FITS + ++	OTHR REFER NONE
RENAL SYMPTOMS	FREQUENCY + ++	DYSURIA + ++	OTHR REFER NONE
OTHER SYMPTOMS			OTHR REFER NONE

SYMPTOMS SUGGESTIVE OF UNWANTED RESPONSES

DROWSY + ++ +++	DEPRESSED + ++ +++	STUFFY NOSE + ++ +++
COLIC + ++ +++	DIARRHOEA + ++ +++	IMPOTENT + ++ +++
WEAKNESS + ++	MUSCLE ACHING + ++ +++	FAILURE EJAC. +

FIRST VISIT ONLY

			600 300 200 100	60 30 20 10	6 3 2 1
ARM CIRCUMFERENCE (cm)					
PLACEBO REACTOR TEST	B.P. BEFORE INJ. (mm.Hg)	SYSTOLIC			
		DIASTOLIC			
	B.P. AFTER INJ. (mm.Hg)	SYSTOLIC			
		DIASTOLIC			

EACH VISIT

BLOOD PRESSURE (mm.Hg)	LYING	SYSTOLIC	600 300 200 100	60 30 20 10	6 3 2 1
		DIASTOLIC			
	STAND'G	SYSTOLIC			
		DIASTOLIC			
FUND:	SLIGT CH'GE	GROSS CH'GE	PAPILL OED'MA	OTHER	REFER NORM

SIGNS OF HEART FAILURE	JVP +	OED EMA	TEND'R LIVER	BASAL CREPS	TRIPLE RHYTM	P.A.H. EMANS
		OTHER	REFER	NEW LESION	NO. EXAM	NORM
SIGNS OF ATHEROMA	ABS'N'T PULSES	BRUITS	ARHY			
		OTHER	REFER	NEW LESION	NO EXAM	NORM
SIGNS OF IMPAIRMENT OF C.N.S.	SPEECH	INTELL	VISION	CRANI NERVES	MOTOR LOSS	SENSE LOSS
		OTHER	REFER	NEW LESION	NO. EXAM	NORM
URINE	600 300 200 100 ALBUMEN NIL TRCE TR+ T+	60 30 20 10 SPECIFIC GRAVITY	6 3 2		
URINE DRUG TEST	POS	NEG	?	NOT DONE		
PHYSICIANS IMPRESSION OF DRUG REC'd	GUANETHIDINE	METHYLDOPA	DON'T KNOW		
TRIAL PHASE (SUCCEEDING PARAGRAPH)					
MEDICATION PRESCRIBED	CODE NO. 6...3...2...1	DAILY DOSE TABLETS 6...3...2...1	NO. DOSES/DAY 6...3...2...1		
PHYSICIAN	A.N.O.	D.W.V.	J.F.D.		

NOTES OR QUERIES ON STOCKTAKE

FIG. 6

There were 16 hand-outs altogether: those not fully reproduced here consist of a bibliography and summaries of actual clinical observations and statistical analyses based upon them. The clinical evaluation form, however, on which the observations were recorded and which could be read directly by the computer is shown in full (Fig. 6), as are the detailed protocol (Fig. 7), the treatment logistics (Fig. 8), the experimental design (Fig. 9) and the intended plan for statistical analysis (Fig. 10).

PROCEDURE

1. Out-patient trial. Patients admitted to hospital only if clinical condition requires it
2. Double-blind: each treatment in two presentations (differing in colour)
3. Drug code held by
   (a) Manufacturers
   (b) Chief Pharmacist, London Hospital
   (c) Trial co-ordinator
4. Two Phases, each of six weeks duration: each patient seen fortnightly. Half patients start on each treatment. All patients cross over treatments in Phase Two
5. Each patient begins on one capsule daily increasing to two after four days if no unwanted responses
6. At subsequent visits dose increased by two capsules per day to maximum of eight per day until adequate control achieved, or unwanted responses occur
7. In the latter case, dose decreased to highest dose previously tolerated and cyclopenthiazide 0.25 mg/potassium chloride 600 mg tablet added
8. If blood pressure not adequately controlled on maximum permitted dose, diuretic added
9. In Phase 3 patient on treatment preferred from Phases 1 and 2; patients seen at least monthly; progress assessed in terms of blood pressure, heart size, ECG and optic fundus
10. Phase 3 to be of 6 to 18 months duration
11. Social worker to visit home during Phase 1, at end of Phase 2, and in middle of Phase 3; to check symptoms, diet, stresses
12. Normal clinical practice obtains; supplementary drugs given if necessary; dangerous reactions or intolerance must lead to withdrawal

FIG. 7

LOGISTICS

1. Capsules to be identical (LHMC DPT definition)* and contain either 12.5 mg guanethidine or 0.2 mg reserpine: half brown, half white
2. Estimated requirements (assuming all patients will receive the same preparation, half in each colour, throughout Phase Three and that each patient will take eight capsules per day for a maximum of 18 months): 150,000 capsules of each colour of each treatment will be required. To avoid deterioration in storage, supply 50,000 of each drug in each colour initially
3. Appropriate serial number entered by physician on treatment card
4. Appropriate drug and colour dispensed by Pharmacy
5. Social worker to collect all proformata and to notify trial controller when reordering necessary

*Joyce (1968)

FIG. 8

EXPERIMENTAL DESIGN

1. Double cross-over comparison of two drugs (reserpine and guanethidine) orthogonal to two colours (brown—B, white—W)
2. Four treatment combinations
3. Each treatment appears twice in random order in block of eight
4. Expected success rate with either treatment: 50% |
5. Useful difference between treatments: 30% | ∴ n=53
6. 2α=0.05;   β=0.05
7. Use n=64, 4×8 blocks per physician

| | **Dr X** | | | | **Dr Y** | | |
Patient No.	Phase 1	Phase 2	Phase 3 (preference)	Patient No.	Phase 1	Phase 2	Phase 3 (preference)
1	W	B	—	41	W	B	—
2	W	B	—	42	B	W	—
3	B	W	—	43	B	W	—
4	B	W	—	44	B	W	—
5	B	W	—	45	W	B	—
6	W	B	—	46	B	W	—
7	B	W	—	47	W	B	—
8	W	B	—	48	W	B	—

REPEAT 3 TIMES

N.B. To preserve blindness for teaching purposes, only the colour code is given here. In later documents, the treatments are coded: R=reserpine, G=guanethidine.

Fig. 9

INTENDED ANALYSES OF TREATMENT DIFFERENCES
A. **NON-PARAMETRIC:** Binomial or X^2

1. Drop-outs
2. Preferences: colour, drug
3. Signs
4. Symptoms
5. Additional drugs

B. **PARAMETRIC:** Analyses of variance —> t-test

1. Systolic pressures at start of Phase 1
2. Systolic pressure changes Phase 1—Phase 2
3. Systolic pressure changes Phase 3
4. Diastolic pressures at start of Phase 1
5. Diastolic pressure changes Phase 1—Phase 2
6. Diastolic pressure changes Phase 3

Fig. 10

I do not contend that this kind of simulation adequately substitutes for on-line experience with a real trial. But if it is repeated with materials from widely differing kinds of trial, it can provide in a short time a repertoire for testing skills that cannot be equalled in a very long period of pre-occupation with real-life trials. Naturally, even the real-life trial controller is extending his knowledge by discussions, by reading the papers of his colleagues and by attending symposia such as this.

It is suggested that the kind of clinical trial workshop described can be a valuable addition to such sources of information because, unlike most others, it involves active participation. With better planning, more time, and eventually perhaps the provision of at least a few alternative strategic pathways so that the group has some control over outcome, the device can become even more valuable.

To this end, the most important hand-out of all is the Final Evaluation Form (Fig. 11).

EVALUATION

1. What other criticisms can be made of the trial design?

2. What criticisms have you of the documents in this hand-out?

3. Have you any comments upon the description of the Clinical Trial Simulation Workshop given in this symposium?

Please send any comments to:

Department of Pharmacology and Therapeutics,
London Hospital Medical College,
Turner Street, London, E.1.

and in particular, comments upon experience acquired with similar teaching experiments in future.

FIG. 11

REFERENCES

MAINLAND, D. (1960). *Notes from a Laboratory of Medical Statistics*. No. 14. New York.

JOYCE, C. R. B. (1968). *Psychopharmacology: Dimensions and Perspectives*, Chap. 7. London: Tavistock.

HOW TO IMPROVE AT CLINICAL TRIALS.

SEARCHING FOR THE SNAGS

J. F. DUNNE

Introduction

The trial used for the simulation exercise described in the preceding chapter did not suffer from a paucity of planning; but, perhaps because it was conceived and performed entirely within a department of clinical pharmacology where investigation of methodology of controlled experimentation is regarded as an important function of the unit, innovation and experimentation were used more freely than is normally possible. In the event the trial proved to be a useful teaching tool, and all involved learned from it.

Trial objectives

A comparison of reserpine and guanethidine in the treatment of patients with uncomplicated, moderate hypertension was chosen because, although strong evidence has been presented (Metropolitan Life Assurance Co., 1959) that life expectation decreases as blood pressure rises, treatment at present carries a commitment to continue therapy indefinitely, a high incidence of unwanted effects and a danger of producing within patients a neurotic involvement with the disease. In consequence there is doubt whether lesser degrees of essential hypertension producing no symptoms merit treatment. A long-term prospective study is needed to compare the progress of such patients treated on diagnosis with others in whom treatment is delayed until symptoms develop or until secondary, clinically-detectable changes occur. This study was planned to compare treatment regimes suitable for such patients. Methyldopa was not included since reports of haemolytic anaemia and warm antibody formulation associated with its use were published just before the trial was launched (Cahal, 1966; Carstairs *et al.*, 1966). The treatments were compared in terms of the patients' preferences as well as in terms of blood pressure response and the incidence of unwanted effects.

Patient selection

A large proportion of the target population of patients do not normally attend hospital departments. In order to conduct a usefully sensitive trial the active cooperation of local general practitioners was sought and 93 were invited to refer patients; 36 acknowledged the letter and expressed support but only 9 referred a total of 27 patient volunteers. Other suitable patients were referred from various sources within the hospital. This unexpected paucity of patients—only 28 who satisfied all the criteria were referred over a period of nine months—raised several problems in experimental design that were solved by extemporising in an unwilling but, it seemed, legitimate manner.

Although both the competing treatments, reserpine and guanethidine, had been widely used as hypotensive agents for several years, no information regarding their relative acceptability to patients and on which to base an estimate of the number of patients required for the trial was found. Had the intention been to establish overall preferences for each treatment only, a sequential method of analysis would have offered clear advantages. But, because other comparisons of the treatment groups were planned, a fixed sample-size design was chosen sensitive enough to demonstrate with reasonable certainty the smallest difference between the two treatments thought to offer therapeutic advantage. A sample size of 64 was selected allowing detection of a true difference in the preference rates between the competing treatments in the ratio 3:4 at the 5 per cent level of significance with a power of 95 per cent.

Progress of trial

The uncertainty concerning the number of patients needed coupled with the subsequent slow rate of admission of suitable patients to the trial prompted the co-ordinator to submit the patients' preferences for each treatment to sequential analysis. Because the initial preferences were predominantly and significantly in favour of reserpine each assessor was asked to admit patients to the first two blocks only of his allocation in the original design. The apparent effect that this decision and certain other incidents had on the course of the trial was a salutary reminder to us that observations ordered in time may not be randomly drawn and a warning that systematic time-related variations may occur within a trial.

The controller chose a closed sequential design with θ (the probability of a preference for the most popular drug) set at 0·8, a power of 0·95 and a significance level of 0·05. When 14 patients had registered a preference, the sequential pathway crossed the boundary of significance favouring reserpine (Fig. 1) and the co-ordinator decided that the last four treatment blocks (two for each of the clinicians in the original design) should be discarded.

This initial trend, however, was not sustained. The pathway moved away from the zone of significance and at the end of the trial it was approaching the boundary defining 'non-significance' (Fig. 2). How might this be explained and what inferences are we allowed to make from such data? It cannot be denied that the initial sequence of preferences for reserpine may merely represent a run against entropy; that chance presented an unrepresentative cluster of patients. But it is equally plausible that the change in the slope of the sequential pathway reflects a real change in the behaviour of either the assessors, the patients or both actually during the course of the trial.

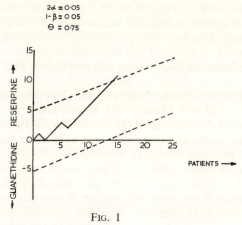

FIG. 1

Sequential pathway after the fourteenth patient had nominated the treatment of choice.

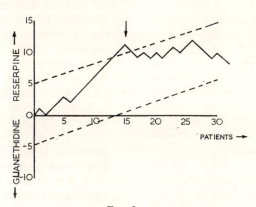

FIG. 2

Sequential pathway at the conclusion of the experiment.

Problems

1. When the clinicians were advised by the controller to cease admissions to the trial they inevitably deduced that one of the treatments was proving more popular. Their conclusion was reinforced by information accidentally received from a pharmacist that stocks of one of the preparations were depleted. Almost simultaneously there was another unfortunate leak of information; the clinicians learned,

again accidentally, from a person working in an ancillary capacity on the trial that, on the basis of their entries on the clinical evaluation forms, they could not reliably distinguish the preparations on clinical grounds. So three events that might have had a bearing on the subsequent development of the trial occurred at the point of inflection on the pathway. The last was particularly unfortunate, for it was far from accurate. It reflected the clinicians impression of the treatment received in only the first four or five preferences that had been made. Subsequently the clinicians' impressions of the treatment received were much more reliable. However, the clinicians were left to believe that they could not identify the treatments, and they could only assume that their influence on the formulation of the preferences, albeit unconscious, might obscure rather than underscore the real superiority of one of the treatments. In other words, if they were completely confused themselves, adding their own confusion to the patients' decision could not possibly sharpen discrimination. So it is possible, although there is no direct evidence for it, that they were less involved from this time in the patients' decisions, and that this change in their attitude towards the formulation of preferences could account for the change of slope of the sequential pathway. Beyond the point of inflection in the pathway there was a relative increase in the popularity of the drug received last by each patient, quite independent of its identity, and this may reflect a less carefully considered judgement caused by the clinician's withdrawal from the decision and an inclination of the patients to avoid a further disruption of their treatment schedule.

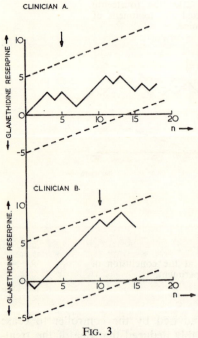

2. But to expose the dangers and limitations of a posteriori reasoning, another explanation of the inflection in this sequential pathway can be provided that is equally convincing. The preferences of the patients seen by each of the two clinicians provide appreciably different slopes on the sequential diagram (Fig. 3). Only patients of clinician B show a

FIG. 3

The preferences of the patients seen by each of the two clinicians.

trend in favour of reserpine and these made the dominant contribution —10 of 14 patients—up to the point of inflection. Because of the uneven rate at which patients of the two clinicians registered their preferences, it is uncertain whether a fundamental difference between the behaviour of the two clinicians or events occurring at the time of the inflection in Figure 2 and the arrows in Figures 3 and 4 are responsible for the change in slope of the pathway.

3. When, instead of drug preferences, the importance of the sequence in which each patient received the drugs is examined, another important discrepancy between the patients supervised by each of the two clinicians is revealed (Fig. 4). A significant majority of the patients of clinician A preferred their second period treatment irrespective of the nature of the drug. (There is no important interaction between the preferred drug and the sequence in which it was given.) In contrast this trend is not evident among the patients seen by clinician B.

The cause of these differences is open to conjecture. Both clinicians were experienced in treating hypertensive patients, both were interested in the methodology of clinical trials and both sought to standardise the way preferences were elicited from the patients. Both were aware of the tendency, when within-patient comparisons are made, of the last treatment to prove more popular than those preceding it.

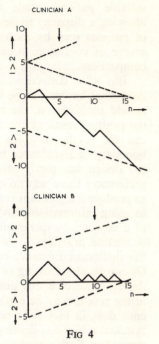

Fig 4

The influence of the sequence in which the treatments were received on the preference of the patients seen by each clinician.

It is possible, although neither clinician wittingly swayed the opinions of his patients, that clinician A was more rigid in his interpretation of the requirement of 'non-intervention' and in his desire to remain impartial was not so persistent in his pressure upon the patients to recall the first period. It is equally possible that clinician B allowed his knowledge of the blood pressure changes and the unwanted effects to influence the patients preferences in a way that was not intended in the design of the trial. But again the alternative possibility exists that the leakage of information that occurred at the points represented by the arrows in Figures 3 and 4 altered the behaviour of both assessors or at least that of clinician A. If such minor factors can decisively alter the pattern of preferences it suggests that, if a real difference between the acceptability of the two treatments does exist, it is not important for most patients.

Discussion

The trial stands open to criticism because the design was changed while it was in progress, but this decision was forced when lack of suitable patients made the original plan unfeasible. Failure in allowing a disparity to develop early in the trial between the numbers of patients seen by each assessor proved to be just as serious as a source of confusion, because it precluded satisfactory inter-observer comparisons.

But what deductions can reasonably be made from these data? And what lessons can be learned from this experience? Which results should be accepted, the negative result of the fixed sample trial or the positive result of the sequential method? Putting it another way, can the results obtained after the sequential pathway crossed the boundary of significance be ignored? Although the choice of sequential design was partly determined by the initial trend of the patients preferences there was no question of deliberately selecting boundaries to produce a significant result. There is no serious theoretical objection to using information provided by early results to fix the boundaries of a sequential experiment and when the sequential t-test is used this is routine practice. So, within the framework of sequential theory, the significant difference between the two treatments is a valid finding. Of course, the crossing of a boundary of significance never indicates the existence of a true difference with certainty; the subsequent trend in the results may be explained on the basis that no important difference does in fact exist between the two treatments. Alternatively, a systematic bias has developed in the experiment that is ' diluting ' the drug effect. Such a possibility clearly exists in this trial.

A striking change in the trend of the results obtained during a trial—and particularly a trend away from a significant difference—may indicate a loss of sensitivity and possible causes for this should be sought. There is no means of knowing how frequently results are compromised in this way, but it is painfully clear that contradictory results occur too frequently in controlled trials and that more effort must be made to analyse inevitable shortcomings. It is irresistible to conclude from this experience that, no matter what form of analysis is finally used, sequential monitoring of the planned comparison and factors liable to introduce bias into the experiment may provide valuable information and that, whenever it seems possible that bias operating from the outset or developing during a trial has obscured a significant difference, the design should be modified and the trial repeated.

Clinical trials are falling into disrepute in some quarters because too often they fail to show any important difference between two treatments when subsequent investigation and a consensus of clinical experience suggest that a real and clinically important difference does, in fact, exist. Controlled comparison must not be rejected as a potentially efficient form of investigation, but the snags must be appreciated. Just as the importance and complimentary nature of statistical and clinical significance are recognised, so must the difference between statistical and clinical sensitivity. All the patients in the world will not give a valid answer to a trial in which there is a serious source of bias.

The fundamental problem in the clinical assessment of drugs is that many factors apart from treatment affect the response of a patient to a disease or affect our interpretation of the progress achieved. Many of these factors operate independently of treatment so there is a built-in hazard in every trial tending to reduce the apparent size of the difference that exists between treatment effects. It would be more appropriate if the error of failing to detect a real and important difference was called an error of the first kind rather than an error of the second kind since this is clearly the prevailing problem. Experiences such as this should alert everyone to search for possible causes of bias in trials with increased rigour.

REFERENCES

CAHAL, D. A. (1966). Methyldopa and haemolytic anaemia (correspondence). *Lancet*, 1, 201.
CARSTAIRS, K., WORLLEDGE, S., DOLLERY, C. T. & BRECKENRIDGE, A. (1966). Methyldopa and haemolytic anaemia (correspondence). *Lancet*, 1, 201.
METROPOLITAN LIFE ASSURANCE COMPANY (1959). Actuarial Statistics.

CONTROLLED TRIALS TO DETECT EFFICACY AND TOXICITY : TRAINING TO MEET TOMORROW'S NEEDS

D. W. VERE

In this paper the broader problems of how to teach and learn the use of clinical trials must be tackled. The most difficult thing in teaching is not to communicate techniques, but to ensure that they will be used with understanding. A trial is only a very useful tool; like any tool its value is sharply defined.

Some common mistakes

There are signs that this is being poorly taught or learned, both for the present and the future use of clinical trials. Two examples should make the point. First, recognition grows that trials may not show up drug toxicity. Chlorpromazine was built in 1950, introduced to anaesthetics the next year and into psychiatry in 1953. The journals for the second half of 1954 make fascinating reading. There are published side by side some of the earliest trials which soundly proved the psychiatric efficacy of the drug, some referring to the occasional case of jaundice but none linking it firmly with the remedy, and letters about the new certainty that these sporadic cases of jaundice were attributable to chlorpromazine (Fig. 1). Had this drug been newly introduced in 1967, Sherlock and Mosteller (1967) agreed that several thousand cases must be observed to detect the incidence of liver damage reliably, for an anaesthetic agent several hundreds of thousands might be needed. Methyldopa is a more striking example. It was known in 1954, shown to lower the blood pressure in 1960, satisfactorily submitted to trials reported in 1961 and found to cause warm antibody formation and haemolysis in 1965. Wintrobe (1968) has delineated a similar story for chloramphenicol; and Doll (1969) recently provided a comprehensive review of many detailed examples.

For these, amongst other reasons, there has been some criticism of clinical trials, and some may even hope that we may join them in wanting to restrict their use. But the fault is not in the trials, which are the only scientific tests of remedies which we possess, but in those who expect too much of them.

A second example is revealed in the attitudes of some journal referees. Recently two controlled trials (not our own) were refused for publication. Whatever may have been the total reasons for rejection, among them were said to be that one trial was single-blind, it being assumed that it should have been double-blind. In the other case a large group of physicians had been asked to state their preferred dose of a remedy; the trial was made at that dose-range but rejected because a referee said the dose was too low to be effective. Neither incident seems to reflect understanding by the referees of the trial as a tool. There are clearly defined cases, infrequent but genuine, where the single-blind trial is a satisfactory tool. The second trial was made not of a drug, but of a fashionable dose range or therapy. The omni-purpose, n-blind, m-dose de rigeur trial, applicable to any and every drug simply does not exist. Why do we have to act as if it does?

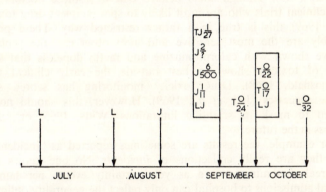

CHLORPROMAZINE
1954 [B.M.J. and LANCET]

FIG. 1

To show that reports of jaundice were largely absent from reports of controlled trials or clinical pharmacological studies.

The strength of trials lies in the flexibility of their design to meet a problem; their success depends upon their design essentials being learnt. The important thing is not so much a grasp of statistical technique as the balanced and critical attitude of mind which gives rise to statistical method and can be learnt from its proper use. Part of this balance is the recognition of how important are psychological factors, which affect those who give and those who take the drugs alike. The papers which follow give striking examples of both effects.

The chief learning needs related to present day clinical trials are summarised in Table I.

TABLE I

Learning needs in relation to present-day clinical trials.

1. Emphasis on balanced design.

2. Accurate recognition of the value and limitations of trials.

3. Psychological factors which affect drug testing, both in the subjects and performers of the tests.

Trials and drug monitoring systems

Some of the limitations of existing clinical trials have been offset by the development of drug toxicity monitoring systems (Finney, 1964; Weir and Crooks, 1966a and 1966b; Slone *et al.*, 1966; Wade and Hurwitz, 1969). Though some believe that it is those doctors who make clinical trials who are most likely to spot incipient drug toxicity (Doll, 1969) this is true in a rather restricted way. These people probably are the most sensitive and alert observers; the problem, as have shown with chlorpromazine and methyldopa, is that some forms of toxicity show up best outside the early clinical trials (Beaconsfield, 1968). Drug toxicity monitoring has scored some notable successes (Jick *et al.*, 1969). However, this should not be allowed to mask its scientific limitations (Witts, 1965) or restrict progress in the future.

For example, the results are sometimes reported as ' incidences ', when they are really collections of *incidents*. No one knows what their real denominators are as yet; certainly events per hundred medical admissions to hospital can only reflect the generality obliquely. When hospital admissions are highly selected, as is usually the case, this amounts to the provision of a false denominator for the incidence fraction, a false security for the investigator and the probablity of false ideas embodied in the matrix of received ' scientific truth '. Drug toxicity monitoring should be regarded as the best expedient available to our present limited resources.

Future developments

What of the future? It seems that there will be a strong need to help both the public, and a future generation of specialists, to learn the meaning of extended controlled trials. Too many people react to the problems of drug development by saying, in effect, ' I want my drugs, I want them cheap, I want them safe, I want them tested, so long as you don't try them first on me '. Education is needed to show people the urgency of responsible collective participation in the testing of new remedies.

With regard to new specialists in clinical pharmacology, it may be possible to predict future needs by projecting our present difficulties forwards. Accepting that trials are limited tools, can a more comprehensive method be foreseen? At present things have settled out into two distinct forms of drug surveillance, the controlled trial (a test of efficacy) and drug toxicity monitoring (a screen for adverse reactions).

Monitored release

Whatever is devised for the future must stand or fall upon whether it conserves the well-founded scientific method which underlies orthodox clinical trial technique, a method which the present divorce between trials and monitoring does not exemplify. It is just possible that a technique, which will be called 'monitored release' of new remedies in this paper, may meet the case. The problem is to find a way to release drugs as easily and safely as possible, while making critical observations of their effects in a far larger group than is possible at present, perhaps 20,000 patients. How can existing principles be projected upon so large a field of study? (Fig. 2).

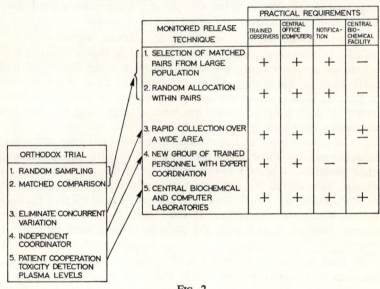

FIG. 2

A projection of orthodox present-day controlled trial techniques towards the practical requirements of future trials.

First, there is the principle of random sampling. It would be possible to enrol pairs of propositi by allocating at random to every p^{th} pair of patients presenting in a defined district either the new remedy or the best available alternative. The practical requirements

17

would be as shown; sufficient trained observers, a good central office and an agreed notification system. Doll (1969) recently discussed the difficulties of notification, but agreed with Finney's suggestion (1964) that N.H.S. prescriptions could give a basis for reliable notification.

The needs for truly comparative data are as shown. Again, reliable notification is the key.

The next principle is the elimination of concurrent variations, including time-dependent effects, which may alter the response to one treatment differently from that to another regime. The practical requirements are met by reliable pairing and rapid recruitment into the trial.

The next principle is that of independence between the trial coordinator and the observers; the nearest approach to 'blindness' possible in large trials. The practical requirement again, is trained personnel.

Lastly, there is detection of patient cooperation, adverse effects and some of the simple measurements of variations in drug metabolism. Here the practical requirements are some central facility to test for drugs and metabolites in urine and plasma, again some agreed compulsory notification scheme, and again trained observers.

This may well seem self-contradictory. Having agreed that controlled trials measure chiefly *efficacy* and fail to detect toxicity, trial techniques are now being invoked to provide some drawn-out and costly form of monitoring. However, there are three strong reasons for this; we must discover not only the frequency of incidents in those exposed to a drug, but also their spontaneous frequencies in a matched population (Reidenberg and Lowenthal, 1968). We need, in other words, a denominator and *two* numerators for each type of clinical incident—one for those given the drug and one for those receiving other remedies. A second reason is to detect delayed alterations in efficacy, as occurred for example with bretylium, ganglion blockers and corticosteroids. Thirdly, we need comparisons of efficacy between regimes which are not confined to the short term. For these reasons, it seems impossible to confine the purpose of long term surveillance to the detection of toxicity.

A final reason for extended monitoring is that it helps in the detection of minority groups within the large numbers recruited to a major trial. Minorities are often submerged in modern trials, so that in effect we tend to select only those remedies which help the majority. This policy (or rather lack of policy) may in the last analysis prove adverse. Remedies may be rejected which help the small groups. The small groups may hold useful genetic characters, though often the reverse is true. At least we are unconsciously affecting our evolution by drugs, and might do well to think about it, at any rate to collect more facts so that we can think about it.

An idealised goal

These practical requirements could summate to the need for what is virtually a new medical auxiliary profession. The thought is less awful than it sounds. Around 1,000 people should be able to collate 10 pairs of propositi each for those drugs which pass a preliminary screen, working in close cooperation with the prescribing doctors who cannot be expected to do this work unaided. Their training should comprise the elements of balanced design, careful record keeping and administration, some knowledge of biochemistry and pharmacy, simple toxicity detection and an awareness of psychological and social factors which affect the testing of drugs. By comparison with other similar professional groups, such training would cost the nation about £3½ M. provided it could be carried on within existing institutions and buildings; some personnel could be drawn from among existing medical and pharmaceutical trainees. The annual maintenance cost might be about two-thirds of this amount. The cost is a relatively small output check upon what is now a £300 M. industrial product per annum, particularly when one recollects the trials and tribulations which it could replace. Clearly, this represents an ideal. It should not be rejected on that account. For example, it would be possible to make a start at once with a small number of selected new drugs. But even the most protean scheme cannot operate unless we begin to train clinical pharmacologists at once.

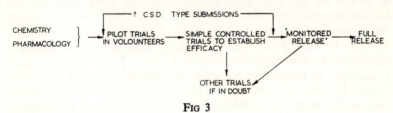

Fig 3

Flow diagrams to contrast the existing, haphazard use of controlled trials in drug release, A, with the proposed system including monitoring release, B.

How would such a scheme change present methods of drug testing? The present situation is shown in Figure 3. Controlled trials may with luck be made by the first interested group to arrive at the scene of the accident or later by a large national organisation, when the dubious drug has irritatingly refused to die from natural causes. Figure 3 also shows a possible monitored release system. Simple trials of ordinary design would be mandatory before public release, to establish whether the new remedy was effective at all. If this trial leaves the matter in doubt, the drug should be submitted to larger orthodox trials before release. (It is to be hoped that in future the nation will be too well informed to allow the rapid release of remedies of slight *efficacy*.) The advantages will be gained by the drug which shows up early as a potential success. Recognising that even repeated orthodox trials cannot be relied upon to reveal toxicity, though they can demonstrate efficacy, the new drug would then be released for prescription, but only on condition that it was submitted to monitored release. Its surveillance would continue, with diminishing elaboration, for about five years. The ethical problem of withholding the new drug from half the tested group is covered by the knowledge that its benefits (and risks) are coming to others several months earlier than at present, and that someone is at least observing what goes on. It would seem at least more responsible to think ahead and appraise the task with realism.

Obviously, the thing would work only in an ideal world where medical men, central and local authorities and industry could trust each other enough to pool some resources for the common good. I believe that such a scheme should not be the direct work of the government, for the social protections of today may become the means of social manipulation of tomorrow (as Joseph showed in Egypt some years ago) and how neatly that could be done with tomorrow's drugs. Also I think that if those whose interest it is to make or test new drugs cannot achieve reliable methods for themselves, in cooperation with official agencies, the job will be done for us by the state. I am implying that we need a new collaborative institute to supervise drug testing, with members drawn perhaps from the Committee on Safety of Drugs, the pharmaceutical industry, and the Royal Colleges and Universities. The alternative is to preserve individual freedom—to meet the chancery of disaster in all its fascinating randomness. Somewhere between these alternatives lies a reasonable balance point. If anyone is displeased, let him suggest something better. I hope that the balance point shall be determined not solely by political, financial or random factors, but also by scientific method with plans to teach the insights of clinical pharmacology, including those psychological factors which influence the evaluation of drugs.

REFERENCES

BEACONSFIELD, P. (1968). Two-tier system for drug testing. *Br. med. J.* **2,** 579.

BINNS, T. B. (1960). Cooperation in drug research. *Glaxo Vol.* **21,** 5.

BINNS, T. B. (1965). The price of therapeutic progress. *Scott. med. J.* **10,** 130.

BINNS, T. B. & BUTTERFIELD, W. J. H. (1964). Clinical trials: some constructive suggestions. *Lancet,* **1,** 1150.

BUTTNER, J. (1966). The detection and evaluation of adverse reactions. *Cronache Farmaceutische,* **5,** 3.

CLUFF, L. E., THORNTON, G., SEIDE, L. & SMITH, J. (1966). Epidemiological study of adverse drug reactions. *Trans. Ass. Am. Phycns,* **78,** 255.

DOLL, W. R. S. (1969). Marc Daniels Lecture to the Royal College of Physicians, London: Recognition of unwanted drug effects. *Br. med. J.* **2,** 69-75.

FINNEY, D. J. (1964). An international drug safeguard plan based on monitoring. *J. chron. Dis.* **17,** 565.

FINNEY, D. J. (1965). The design and logic of a monitor of drug use. *J. chron. Dis.* **18,** 77.

JICK, H., SLONE, D., WESTERHOLME, B., INMAN, W. H. W., VESSEY, M. P., SHAPIRO, S., LEWIS, G. P. & WORCESTER, J. (1969). Venous thromboembolic disease and ABO blood type. *Lancet,* **1,** 539-541.

REIDENBERG, M. M. & LOWENTHAL, D. J. (1968). Adverse non-drug reactions. *New Engl. J. Med.* **279,** 678, and annotation (1959). *Br. med. J.* **1,** 798.

SHERLOCK, S. & MOSTELLER, (1967). Discussion of chapter by Sherlock, S. on Drugs and hepatotoxicity. In *Drug Responses in Man,* p. 153. Ed. Wolstenholme and Porter, Ciba Symposium.

SLONE, D., JICK, H., BORDA, I., CHALMERS, T. C., FEINLEIB, M., MUENCH, H., LIPWORTH, L., BELLOTTI, C. & GILMAN, B. (1966). Drug surveillance utilising nurse monitors: an epidemiological approach. *Lancet,* **2,** 901.

WADE, O. L. & HURWITZ, N. (1969). Intensive hospital monitoring of adverse reactions to drugs. *Br. med. J.* **1,** 531-535.

WEIR, R. L. D. & CROOKS, J. (1966a). *Med. Rec.* **7,** 311.

WEIR, R. L. D. & CROOKS, J. (1966b). *Med. Rec.* **8,** 7.

WINTROBE, M. M. (1968). The therapeutic millenium and its price. *J. R. Coll. Phycns, Lond.* **3,** 99.

WITTS, L. J. (1965). Adverse reactions to drugs. *Br. med. J.* **2,** 1081.

INDEX

251

Printed at The Central Press, Belmont St., Aberdeen.